T0370506

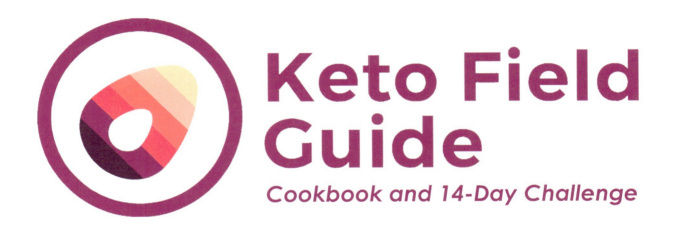

Keto Field Guide

Cookbook and 14-Day Challenge

Breanna Reeser

AuthorHouse™
1663 Liberty Drive
Bloomington, IN 47403
www.authorhouse.com
Phone: 1 (800) 839-8640

Published by AuthorHouse 10/30/2018

ISBN: 978-1-5462-6447-7 (sc)
ISBN: 978-1-5462-6448-4 (e)

Library of Congress Control Number: 2018912325

Print information available on the last page.

Any people depicted in stock imagery provided by Getty Images are models,
and such images are being used for illustrative purposes only.
Certain stock imagery © Getty Images.

This book is printed on acid-free paper.

Because of the dynamic nature of the Internet, any web addresses or links contained in
this book may have changed since publication and may no longer be valid. The views
expressed in this work are solely those of the author and do not necessarily reflect the views
of the publisher, and the publisher hereby disclaims any responsibility for them.

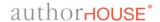

Author Bio

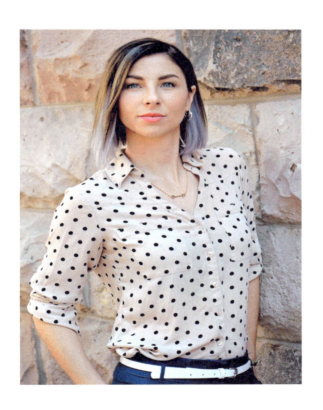

Dr. Breanna Reeser is an exercise physiologist and health behavior change specialist with 10 years of experience in preventative wellness and chronic disease management. She consults with healthcare providers and executive groups to improve techniques for facilitating health behavior and lifestyle changes. She also guest lectures on the science behind behavior change methods at universities and conferences internationally. She was awarded a scholarship through Arizona State University (ASU) and United States Agency for International Development (USAID) in fall of 2017 to complete her dissertation data collection in hospital systems throughout Southeast Asia. As a part of her research, she conducted an Integrated Healthcare needs assessment and consulted on quality improvement for disease management for hospital systems in Chiang Mai, Thailand.

Welcome to your 14-day guide to resetting your metabolism and reaching your best health. Ketogenic eating can be intimidating, but SSOHealth is bringing you an easy solution with our *Ketogenic Field Guide*. Get up to speed on ketosis basics with our carefully curated FAQs and enter a state of ketosis quicker with less hassle by following our meal plan, grocery list and recipes! Challenge yourself and track your progress through the 14 daily journal pages and meditations. Want to join our fast-growing online community for more support? Join our Keto Field Guide All Access E-Pass!

The All Access E-Pass gives you an invitation to be a part of a virtual community where people just like you are making healthy choices in their lives using high fat nutrition. This is a great long-term solution to your busy and complex life. The All Access E-Pass is full of informative videos on a private YouTube channel, curated and vetted recipes on a private Pinterest board, and chances to win prizes through our quarterly challenges hosted on a private Facebook group. All content is updated regularly for you to participate in, pull from, and contribute to at your pace. Access to is managed on one easy to use sign-in page. To sign up for the KFG All Access E-Pass, go to www.ketofieldguide.com.

Thank you to our sponsor and partnership with SSOHealth, who offers custom health coaching solutions for ketosis and also for health, fitness and exercise goals of all kinds.

"What will you be able to accomplish when you reach your best health?"

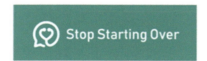 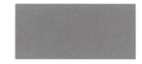

www.SSOHealth.com
~Where Fitness is a Mindset & Exercise is Medicine! ~

Table of Contents

Introduction

My relationship with food has been all over the map. I have been everything from a binge eater to raw vegan and back again, all in the name of health. I recognize that some of my choices surrounding diet have been for health decisions, while others have been out of fear, ignorance, or vanity. I have not always treated my body right and I have even used health techniques in such unhealthy ways that I harmed my body. The bottom line is that knowing exactly what to eat is hard, even for a person who has devoted their career to health behaviors. There is a lot of information out there, most of it conflicting and not all of it truthful. No one can tell you exactly what to eat for a specific outcome, although they will tell you they can. We are all different and what will work for some won't work for others. Hell, what worked for me years ago does not work for me now, and I bet you can relate. Food landscapes change, ingredients change, our bodies needs will change, and even our cultural and social needs change. There are a lot of things that go into choosing a meal, so if you are reading this right now and you are nervous and wondering if you are making the right decision, I am here to tell you that you are in good company. No one specific diet will "fix" you. No one product or habit will get you entirely to your goals. In fact, it is not even about that. Eating and the relationship we have with our food and our bodies should be about finding a balance to feel the best we can feel in the time we have so that we can do the things that make us happy. Eating should be about fueling your body with nutrition so that you can walk your daughter down the aisle, take that trip with your besties, celebrate your anniversaries, and physically do the things that bring meaning to your life. Food should fuel your adventures.

Right now, you are choosing to embark on a 14-day journey of eating a certain way in hopes of changing your body for the better. You will be challenged to think about your relationship with food and to break through barriers you have been holding onto for years. You will be challenged to recognize the truths and lies in food marketing, and hopefully, you will begin to be a consumer of real foods for a lifetime of health and wellness. Eating ketogenic foods for 14-days will be an experience. It may not change your life, but it certainly could. Choosing to commit to 14-days of healthy mindset, healthy eating, and positive intention is surely a great start to the rest of your healthy life.

How Ketosis Chose Me

I was first introduced to the idea of high-fat nutrition while working on a research project in Southeast Asia. I am an exercise physiologist and I make my living by helping people design exercise programs to manage their diseases like diabetes and heart disease. I also create exercise programs for athletes to improve performance and succeed in events like marathons. While in Asia, I met and spoke with athletes who have used ketosis as a way to improve their performance in a variety of sports and athletic events. I was initially and immediately opposed to this idea but was also confronted by the lack of understanding that I had on the topic. I had not read any research or even tried this technique out myself, so I effectively knew nothing about the process or the impact on the body or on performance. I certainly did not know why keto seemed to work for these people, or if it could work for anyone else. Fortunately, I had recently developed a new practice of recognizing and rejecting any of my reactions that may be social or culturally constructed (if you do not have this as a regular practice I highly recommend it). Regularly scrutinizing my reactions and thought-constructions on any topic for authenticity has helped me break through otherwise limiting patterns of thought that do not serve me or others. This seemed like one of the times to dig a little deeper into a topic in did not understand. As a result, I recognized that this immediate opposition I had may be shortsighted and unfounded. Right then I decided to do two things; research the topic before making a judgement, and test drive this diet myself.

I was challenged during my research. There were a few concepts that I struggled with at first, concepts like not being able to eat fruit, eating saturated fats, and not having enough carbohydrates to fuel muscle action. Yes, I hear you, and I totally agree with you that cutting out an entire food group sounds crazy and not at all balanced or healthy. Trust me, I missed, craved, and pined for apples during my first few weeks on ketosis, but then it got easier, and I survived. Once you become keto-adapted (covered later in the book) you can add in certain low-carb fruits like berries without kicking you out of the fat for energy system of ketosis. You can also cycle off ketosis, which is highly recommended for long-term success, and have meals with carrots and potatoes every once in a while. It is amazing how much appreciation you will have for the natural carbs in your diet once you begin this journey. I remember the pure ecstasy of eating a raspberry after being completely carb-free for one month. I stood over the carton of raspberries and popped one into my mouth. Suddenly my eyes went wide, and that pleasure sensor in my brain went into overdrive. I started making some pretty embarrassing sounds, gushing over how amazing the taste was. Does this sound familiar to anyone reading who has done keto diets before? I looked over at my perplexed and slightly concerned husband and said something along the lines of "OMG is this just me or is this the best raspberry bunch we have ever had, like 100 times more sweet than usual?" And with a furrow in his brow, he said, "Yup, it's just you." I had actually reset my taste sensors after a month of extremely limited carbohydrates to appreciate natural sweetness again. Amazing.

I dug into the topics that concerned me and tried to understand them fully. I couldn't in good conscious recommend this style of eating if I was against some of the principals of the theory. It turns out that there are some common misconceptions about the diet. In my ten years of exercise programming for weight loss to injury rehabilitation and performance enhancement, I have always advocated for plant-based diets rich in leafy greens. I had it in my mind that you couldn't have a plant-based leafy green diet while in ketosis. That is way off. In fact, it is crucial that people on ketosis work hard to incorporate greens and vegetables into their diet as a part of the micronutrient content every day. Similarly, you do not have to stuff your face with protein as you might expect. Ketosis is way more concerned with having high-quality fats and about the ratio of fat to carbohydrates than it is with the amount of protein you consume. In fact, consuming too much protein could inhibit your body from reaching full positive effects. Having a moderate protein intake, ultra-low carbohydrate intake and a very high fat intake will support the best function your body can manage.

As I began to research and prepare for my biohacking experiment, I started to reinforce truths that I had already known and even coached on, things like the dangers and misguidance of the FDA food label. The food industry has done a fantastic job of confusing us and misguiding our health efforts to sell more poor quality products. Take the low-fat diet crazes for example. Low-fat products are a scam. I don't mean foods that are naturally low in fat; I mean products that have been modified to be low fat. Low-fat foods tend to be full of hidden added sugars. The chances are that most of the low-fat packaged foods are modifications of full-fat, saturated fat animal products like yogurts, creams, and milk. Producers will chemically remove fats and then replace them with added sugar and salt to enhance the flavor. Low-fat products with chemically enhanced flavors are killing us, contributing to the high epidemic of heart diseases, obesity, diabetes and metabolic syndromes. Please, don't take my word for it, next time you are out grocery shopping check the labels. Put the low fat and full-fat products side by side and see what the sugar and salt contents are. Never mind the calories, start to train your brain to think in value instead of quantity. What is the nutritional value of the foods you are eating?

Healthy fat intake from plant-based sources like avocado, nuts, olives, and coconut are all health promoting and do not contribute to metabolic syndromes like obesity. Fat takes a little longer to process, so the slow release of energy into the system does not cause spikes in blood sugar, making this an excellent option for diabetic and pre-diabetic patients that struggle with stabilizing their blood sugars. Plant-based fats also do not contribute to high cholesterol levels! On the contrary, American Heart Association recognizes high HDL levels (plant-based fats and fish oil) as negative correlations to heart disease and stroke. That means eating more high-fat foods from plant sources lower your risk of high cholesterol and heart disease.

Foods high in the right fats are wonderfully nutritious and support brain and organ function, while foods with added sugars and fake sugars are terribly inflammatory and damaging. Even recent publications on saturated fats show that prior studies flagging saturated fats as harmful are inconclusive at best. I asked these four questions and looked to published and peer-reviewed research to answer them;

1. Is there enough research to support the notion that saturated fat correlates to heart disease? Answer: Studies found no statistical significance of reducing saturated fats to reduce heart attacks, strokes or all-cause deaths.
2. Is there research to support the medical use of high-fat diets (including saturated fat) to treat epilepsy? Answer: Yes
3. Is there research to support the notion that excessive use of sugar in the diet contributes to disease, inflammation and poor health? Answer: Yes (recommended daily intake from CDC and FDA is 33 grams or lower)
4. Does eating fat make you fat or sick? Answer: Nope! Eating fat DOES NOT make you fat! Eating fats while cutting out carbs causes your body's energy system to run smoother, burning more fat while giving you energy!

That is as far as I will dive into the science or research with you in this book. There are significant and reliable resources on the science and study of high-fat nutrition that I have listed in the back of the book for your reference, and I urge you to look at them if you are interested. For our purposes here in this book and guide, we will stick to the practical and real-life application of how ketosis has helped many people reach their goal weights and reset their metabolism, and how it can work for you as well.

My Ketosis Story

I began ketosis all in after spending about a month researching the topic. My reasons for starting ketosis were many. As I mentioned, one of the biggest reasons for starting this diet was to vet it for a client of mine, but as I began to research this for my own use, I became more and more excited to try it out. Experts on the topic advertise one specific side effect that I couldn't wait to experience, improved brain function. Many people who get into ketosis experience a very clear and productive mental capacity, above and beyond anything they have ever experienced before, and I wanted in on that more than anything else. Another enticing side effect advertised was decreased anxiety and improved GI function, both things I was desperately in need of. I was just coming home to the United States after a particularly grueling, emotional, and trying research placement in Thailand. While in Thailand I was struggling with depression from being away from my family and immense stress from collecting data that would soon become my dissertation for my Doctorate. I was battling barriers in culture and language while taking 800 level courses online from the US and carrying out a research project in multiple hospitals. My stress and anxiety ultimately lead to an ulcer and some weight gain. When returning home, I was resolved to do something natural to repair my health and take care of myself. So, on December 8th, 2018 I went "keto". What you should know about me is that I do not have an addictive personality and although I sincerely empathize and work with people who do have these struggles, I never have firsthand felt the addition of a specific food. You should also know that when I resolve to do something, I strive to make it as mentally easy to accomplish as possible. I tell myself daily, sometimes constantly minute by minute, that I do not miss the things I am leaving behind and that I am utterly happy with my current diet. This mindset makes it incredibly easy to change when I want to. Someone comes up to me with a cookie (and I LOVE chocolate chip cookies!), I will powerfully say, no thanks I do not want that because I am loving my body right now and that cookie is literally poisonous. Doughnut? Poisonous. Cupcake for a coworker's birthday? No thanks, Poisonous. Free soda for Employee Appreciation Day? NOT TODAY SATAN. POISONOUS! It is obnoxious and hilarious. Just the reaction I get from some people gives me both joy and entertainment. That practice is not for everyone, but it really helps me. It helps me to hear my voice say those things out loud. It helps to reinforce my decisions, and it helps to call out the lack of nutrition in those items. Sure, it will be okay to partake in those things once in a while, but not now. Wait until you have completed the challenge and you have kicked your sugar habit. When you have committed to a challenge to change your eating habits, it is incredibly important to follow through. You are worth it.

I spent 14-days on a strict ketosis diet with only 5% or less of my daily intake of nutrients representing total (not net) carbohydrates; literally the only carbohydrates I consumed in those first two weeks came from broccoli and kale. I drank lots and lots of herbal tea, an occasional diet soda, and electrolyte enhanced water. My diet was very basic and simple, which worked well for me due to my busy schedule and, lets just call it what it is, my lack of motivation to cook. I spent months in Asia eating fresh fruit and cheap street food with no option to cook my own meals, I hardly wanted to come back to the U.S. and slave away for hours on elaborate Pinterest dishes. That used to be my thing, but priorities change and now I don't get as much value from preparing food as I once used to. If that sounds like you, I have an option that you will love; My exact meal plan for those two weeks can be found under "No-Cook Busy/Lazy Keto Options". For everyone who still loves to get their hands dirty for a great and beautiful meal, we have those too.

After those first 14-days, I was hooked on how great I looked, performed and felt so I kept going. I ended up staying in ketosis for over two months with only one "cheat" day (and during the holidays too!). I felt fantastic, my digestive health was amazing; no more bloated feeling, nausea or embarrassing gas from my ulcer. I ended up losing about 12 pounds, down lower than my high school weight, without reducing my caloric intake or feeling hungry at all. I did, and still do, feel the mental clarity that was advertised as well as the amazing energy and drive. I didn't struggle with keto flu (addressed later in the book) at all, and I attribute the lack of crummy feelings during that transition to a specific regimen of supplements I took (also addressed later in the book and highly recommended). I did not feel much reduction in anxiety, but I better save that topic for a whole different book, time and place.

At the same time, I started ketosis; I also started to practice yoga more regularly and to challenge my physical body more. I realized that my joints didn't flare up after yoga sessions like they had (even the right kneecap that I have been nursing for over a year started to feel "normal" during practices) and that when I tried new poses above my scope of practice, I routinely got injured less. Before ketosis, if I were to try a handstand and fall out of it, I would inevitably end up with some sort of muscle strain, but now I could try a few times, fall a few times, laugh at my own mistakes and never experience a strain at all. This improvement alone was worth ditching the carbs. As a result of this change, my yoga practice became stronger, my body became stronger, my enthusiasm and passion for life grew stronger, and my self-confidence became stronger.

I have now participated in a few cycles of ketosis and continued to stay keto-adapted for over six months. I had such huge successes with my experiment that I started to talk to more people about it, recommending it clinically in my professional practice and socially with my friends and family.

From personal success to shared success

February 2018, I guided my first group of 10 people through a 14-day prescriptive diet challenge for ketosis. The group was a mixed bag with most people generally healthy and only wanting to lose a few pounds. The results were incredible with the most weight loss at 12 pounds in the 14-days. The average weight loss during the challenge was four pounds in 14-days. Clients reported a reduction in joint pain, improved sleep, improved mental clarity, improved blood sugar levels for diabetics, and no real hunger feeling while on the challenge. The challenge was not without issues though. Some also reported constipation, low energy until day 4-7, low energy in the afternoons, and intense carb cravings for the first four days. Everyone is a little different and will experience this challenge a little differently.

Since that first group, I have personally coached people through the process and have refined the challenge based on excellent feedback from real experiences. Now I am sharing with you a tried and true method to get into ketosis fast and reset your body's metabolism to reduce weight and improve health in just 14-days. If you are excited to see what 14-days of ketogenic eating can do for you, let's get started!

A note about SSOHealth Coaching:

If you are reading this book and I have not had the pleasure or opportunity to first talk with you about the ketogenic diet and benefits, I urge you to reach out to me, or at the very least connect with me on some sort of social media. There is a lot of information out there, much of which is contradictory or even downright untrue. I know that making a big change in lifestyle is incredibly taxing, emotionally and sometimes physically. I find that the people who do the best on this challenge and with this change are the ones who are connected to a resource that they can trust. You have a few options from SSOHealth to support you on your keto journey. Hop over to the website, blog, Instagram, and Facebook page for free content that will keep you motivated, interested, supported, and educated on ketogenic foods. Then, if you want a little more support, sign up for our newsletter and join our private VIP group. Next, if you want personalized help to reach your specific goals, schedule a telephonic appointment with me and we can hash it out together. All of this can all be found on the website at www.ssohealth.com !

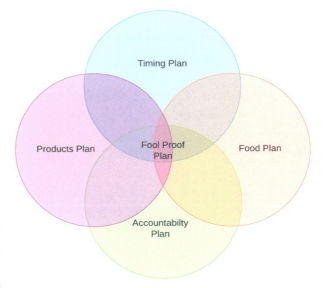

Getting Started

Plan for Success

Planning in advance and having a few great backup plans for unforeseen events will always make any challenge much easier. This is especially true when starting a new diet or exercise program. Planning for this challenge will include these four pillars of a fool-proof plan; Timing, Food, Products, and Accountability. Being intentional about these four areas will ensure that you hit your goals with the least amount of risk for failure.

Four Pillars of Success

–   **Timing:** At least a week before you start the 14-day challenge, make sure to review the entire book and all the recommendations. When will you start your challenge? A weekday, a weekend? Are there any holidays, birthdays, or other social events during this time? Will you have enough time to prepare meals and read the daily entries? When will you prepare meals; what day and time? When will you read the daily entries; before bed, on a lunch break or right when you wake up? Being intentional about timing and committing to a timing plan can remove many barriers to success. Our recommendation when planning for timing is to grocery shop on Saturday and then meal prep on Sunday for a start date of Monday.

- **Food:** What meal plan will you follow? Will you follow the exact 14-day meal guide and recipes to the last detail? This will give you the best results, but it is not the only option. For example, you may want to follow the no-cook plan a few days a week or you may want to sub in a pescatarian meal for one or two of your dinners. If so, you will have to modify your grocery list and plan accordingly. Will you have any meals during this week that you will eat at a restaurant? If so, check the restaurant guide at the back of this book and make sure to check the restaurant menu in advance to plan for what you will order.

- **Products:** There are a few products that I recommend and use as a part of my ketogenic experience. You do not have to use them, but in my experience, they make a very big difference. You will need to decide now if you will take a supplement or not and which supplements/products you will take or use. If you are going to use a product, where will you get it from? How long will it take to receive it? If ordering online, make sure to order 5-7 days in advance. Products we recommend are:

    1. <u>Ketone Urine Sticks</u>- Keto sticks are urine test strips that allow you to recognize if you are producing ketones in your body. This is a good indicator of whether or not you are in ketosis and how far into ketosis you are in. Find the test strips we use on www.ketofieldguide.com

    2. <u>Exogenous Ketones</u>- This is a commercial product that introduces ketones into the body from an outsides source, meaning that your body does not have make them to have the good and positive effects of having ketones. This has been very helpful for me, especially in those first few days when your body is transitioning from a carbohydrate energy system to a fat for fuel energy system. Your body will take a few days to burn all the existing carbs and start to produce ketones. Think of this product as a bridge between the two energy systems. Just throw a scoop into your bulletproof coffee every A.M. and feel the energy and mental clarity flow! This is how I completely skipped feeling the dreaded "Keto Flu". My favorite product is Chocolate Sea Salt by Perfect Keto.

    3. <u>Fat Supplement</u>- Often people find it hard to get the right amount of fat into their daily diet. One way to supplement this is to take a fat supplement. Caprylic acid supplements are also useful for digestive issues and ulcers. Take two capsules 2 x a day to kick up the fats and give your body the extra fuel it craves.

4. Electrolyte Supplement- While the last three products were optional, we highly recommend that you take an electrolyte supplement while in ketosis. Fruit is a major source of many electrolytes in our diet, so cutting them out completely will leave you deficient. Finding a sugar free or low sugar electrolyte supplement can be difficult. Our favorite is Vega Sport Electrolyte Hydrator with zero calories and no fake sugar. This one also has copper and zinc! If you do not want to take this supplement, consider taking a pill supplement like magnesium and calcium. You can drink water fortified with electrolytes or try another sugar free option. Remember to check the label for hidden ingredients!

— **Accountability:** Will someone be joining you in this challenge? We highly recommend that you invite someone, or a few friends to join your challenge with you. It is easier, and more fun, to stick to a challenge when you have a buddy to talk to about the successes and challenges. SSOHealth also offers a private VIP challenge group as a part of the KFG All-Access E-Pass. Challenges take place four times a year. As a part of this group you will have a community who is going through the challenge with you each time. They also offer customized coaching for the two-week challenge that has been shown to greatly improve success.

Take the time to answer all of the questions outlined in the Four Pillars of Success. The answers to these questions become your personal success plan. Once you have your plan in place, it is time to put in the preparation work.

Preparation Check-list

☑ I have read through the book, including recipes, meal plans, and getting started sections.

☑ I have walked through and written down my plan for success, including when I will start this challenge, when I will grocery shop, when I will meal prep, what exactly I will eat, which products I will use, and who I will do the challenge with.

☑ I have purchase and received all products I will use.

☑ I have designated an accountability partner and/or completed my first call with my coach.

Choosing a timeframe to complete the challenge

- Choose periods of low stress and low risk of unforeseen events
- Take into account holidays, birthdays, and other carb-filed celebrations
- Make sure you have time before the start of the challenge to read and process all information
- Make sure you have time to plan, purchase food and prep food each week

High-fat Nutrition FAQs

Welcome to the frequently asked questions of keto. This section is meant to anticipate and answer your questions concisely and clearly without overwhelming you. The answers to each of these questions are based on a combination of professional experience and research. Once you have read through this section you should have a great foundational understanding of ketosis and ketogenic eating that you can continue to build upon throughout the challenge. If you find that you are struggling with concepts or have more questions left unanswered, reach out to us on our social media for clarity.

The Basics:

This challenge is not a product driven experience. I am not trying to sell you on a single product or solution. This is an educational experience where you will learn about food, about how your body uses food, and how to provide your body with quality food to improve your health. You will feel challenged to think differently and to break your addiction to sugars (both processed and natural forms of sugar). The next two weeks will focus on real and fresh foods that you can purchase on your own in the grocery store. The food in this challenge is real nutrition that you can control and replicate on your own for years to come. Use this challenge and this book to create a new foundation of what achieving health through nutrition can be like for you. Let's start with some of the basic questions and answers that you may have.

1. What Is "Keto"?

The term "keto" is used to signify a type of diet used in health, wellness, and weight loss. The word keto is short for the word ketosis, a state in which your body starts to produce ketones as a byproduct of using fat for fuel. Ketosis happens when you stop eating carbs and start eating high amounts of healthy fats. It may seem concerning at first, but the science behind this diet is well documented. Wading through the media onslaught of food marketing is difficult, especially when most of what we see says to eat low fat and supports the use of added sugars. The Keto Field Guide does not explore the science behind the use of ketosis; rather we strive to provide a method and framework for putting the science into practice. We encourage you to do the research on the "why" of ketosis outside of this book if you are interested and still have questions regarding that aspect.

"keto" or "ketosis" is often used as a medical diagnosis for a critical state that Type 1 Diabetics can get into if they do not have enough available glucose in their body. For these people with T1D, ketosis is a life-threatening emergency, so when some people hear "keto," they automatically think bad health. However, that is far from accurate. For people with healthy functioning metabolisms (and for T2 Diabetics), the act of voluntarily feeding your body fat for fuel will put your metabolism in a state of dietary ketosis without the risk of critically low available energy. When you think of keto, think about it as an efficient way to feed your body with a diet that is very high in fats and very low in sugars (or carbs). This is very important; to be in ketosis and get the benefit of the experience, you MUST NOT have any available sugar in your system that your body can use as fuel. Think of it as switching your engine onto premium gasoline.

2. What Are the Benefits?

There are multiple benefits of being on a ketogenic diet. The most significant advantage that most people see with this diet is weight loss, but it is more than just that. Many athletes and revolutionary thinkers use the state of ketosis to kick-start their health, make their bodies more efficient, and promote brain function. Research on ketogenic eating shows improvements in many chronic conditions including stabilizing blood sugars, reducing inflammation, improving energy and decreasing stress. Tim Ferriss also talks about how he treated his Lyme disease with ketosis on his podcast, and Dr. Joseph Mercola speaks about ketosis prevention and a possible cure for most cancers.

3. How Can I Tell If I am In Ketosis?

Being in ketosis is an "all or nothing" kind of thing. Either your body is using sugar for fuel, or your body is using fat for fuel, there is no "in-between." When your body uses fat for fuel, the byproduct is ketones. There are two main ways to test for ketones, blood levels with a finger stick or urine levels with a dip stick. The urine level test kit is affordable and minimally invasive. You can find it on the website at www.ketofieldguide.com. Truly being in ketosis is a great goal, but not the real point of this 14-day challenge, and certainly not the point of the transformation you will hopefully undergo way beyond these 14-days. More importantly than asking "Am I in ketosis?" Is to ask, "Have I changed my relationship with food to become more nutrition/health centered and less emotional?"

4. Are There Risks Involved?

Like anything new, there may be risk involved. There is a very minimal risk for specific medical conditions and even lower risk for generally healthy people. Always consult your doctor if you have any diagnoses or any questions (and see the medical FAQs). There are adverse side effects (keto flu) while your body is transitioning to the new energy system.

5. How Long Should I Stay on a Ketogenic Diet?

This is a highly personal decision. There are no negative side effects of being in a state of ketosis other than electrolyte depletion that you can manage with a supplement. Many people who eat in this style for medical purposes stay in ketosis for months. As your body learns to adapt to using fat as an energy source, you will easily be able to incorporate more healthy carbohydrates into your diet occasionally and may benefit from a slow carbohydrate day here and there where you shoot for 20% of your macros from healthy carbohydrates. You should not stay on traditional ketosis macro splits if you are trying to lift heavy to build muscle. In this instance, adding in carbs at the right times will benefit your goals more than staying under 25 grams of carbohydrates will.

6. Does Eating Fat Make You Fat?

Short answer, nope!

Eating fat DOES NOT make you fat!
Eating fats while cutting out carbs makes your
body's energy system run smoother,
burning more fat while giving you energy!

7. What Happens If I Mess Up and Eat Carbs?

Here is the hard conversation. You are either in a state of burning fat for fuel or you are not. If you eat almost correct and miss ketogenic state by a centimeter, it might as well be a mile. Commit to the time frame to give your body the chance to make it into ketosis. This decision will take willpower and assertive choices; even a few extra carbs will make the difference between feeling sluggish on keto and feeling fantastic energy while losing weight and performing better. Don't cheat; you deserve better!

8. Can Ketosis Help Me Lose Weight?

All recent research supports caloric deficit as the only way to reduce weight. This means that science shows that it does not matter if you eat Paleo, keto, Adkins, or shitty, as long as you burn more than you take in, you will lose weight. While this is absolutely true, this does not take into account the performance of the body and how nutrition affects body systems. If you eat 1200 calories of nutritious and bioavailable foods, you will feel different than if you take in 1200 calories of doughnuts. Eating empty processed foods will make you sluggish, tired, bloated, irritable and hungry. Eating ketogenic with high fat nutrition will make you feel satiated, balanced, lighter, and energized. In the long run, it is more sustainable to eat fewer calories of nutrient-dense foods than it is to eat fewer calories in a standard processed diet. Eating ketogenic will allow your body to find a healthier weight naturally with nutrition, and you may find that you need less calories as a result. So, long answer, yes, but not in the way that you may have expected.

9. What do I Do After my Keto Challenge Ends?

Keep connected and keep in touch through our All-Access E-Pass! Coming off of ketosis and reintroducing carbohydrates into your diet can be a scary process. This process will depend on you and what your goals are. Some of you may feel great at the end of this challenge and choose to continue with this style of eating. I say go for it! If you do decide to reintroduce carbohydrates, now is the time to set a foundation of what you will allow in your body. Healthy carbs from fruits and vegetables can be very beneficial, but returning to processed, refined carbohydrates like bread and pasta will likely make you feel ill and gain weight. Choose your cheat meals so that you are living a full and balanced life, but keep in mind the type of life you want to lead. When your body is fueled with high-quality nutrition, there will be no end to the possibilities for your health.

The Nutrition:

The most important aspect of achieving ketosis is eating the correct foods. Fueling your body with fats is how you achieve the ketosis state and start to reap the benefits. During this challenge, and when you choose to be in ketosis, you will give up fruit and lots of vegetables (except for the occasional berry). That does not mean that fruit is inherently bad, it just means that for this style of eating, you will not eat them. Again, cycling in a day or two of slow carbs (like fruits and starchy vegetables) will be beneficial once you become keto adapted and after you have participated in the 14-day challenge. Let's cover some of the common nutrition questions and answers about ketosis.

1. What Can I Eat on Keto?

Fats, any animal proteins, and any leafy greens. The keto diet consists of high-fat, low-carb, nutrient-dense foods. Around 75% of your intake should be healthy fats such as olive oil, coconut oil, butter, palm oil and some nuts and seeds. Fat is essential in the ketogenic diet because it is what fuels the body and prevents hunger and fatigue. You should also consume a variety of non-starchy vegetables such as brussels sprouts, asparagus, broccoli, cucumber, and all sorts of leafy greens. In more moderate amounts you should intake foods that are high in protein and low in carbs. This includes bone-broth, meat, fish, eggs, poultry, and full-fat dairy products. Stay away from any sugar, processed foods, all grains, and starchy vegetables. As always, drink plenty of water.

2. How is Keto Different from Atkins/Paleo?

Lots of things are different! Keto is a high fat moderate protein diet, it is not a high protein diet. Atkins and Paleo do not have the same high fat intake that is necessary to change how your body makes energy. Ketogenic eating can be considered a refined version of Paleo, focusing on eliminating grains and improving the quality of the food you eat.

3. What are Macros, What Should They Be, and How Can I Track Them?

Macronutrients are the basic building blocks of food and can be broken down into three categories: Fats, Carbohydrates, and Proteins. These are typically measured in grams. The amount in grams of macronutrients needed to consume on a ketogenic diet may vary for each person, but it is crucial to measure the percentage of each in your whole diet. For ketosis, the break down should be 70-80% Fats, 20-30% Protein, and less than 8% Carbs. We recommend that you find a solution to track your macros that works for you. A few options we like include MyFitnessPal and Ketoned (an app coming soon).

4. Are There Good Fats and Bad Fats?

There *are* bad fats, but it will probably surprise you. Saturated fats are GOOD fats. There is no substantial evidence that saturated fats contribute to heart disease! Bad fats include processed, refined oils (vegetable oil, corn oil, etc.).

5. Do I Need to Take Supplements to get into Ketosis?

While not completely necessary, some supplements will be helpful to kickstart your ketosis and ward off any symptoms you may feel in the process of transitioning energy systems. We recommend a Medium Chain Triglyceride (MCT) supplement, exogenous ketones, and a sugar-free or low-carb electrolyte solution. See our recommendations in the plan for success section.

Healthy Fats:
Avocado, Coconut Oil, Clarified Butter, Olive Oil
Pistachios, Pecans, Walnuts, Almonds
Cheese, Eggs, Fish, Grass-Fed Meats

6. Can I be Vegan or Vegetarian and Still Get into Ketosis?

Yes, but the food options will be even more restricted. If you eat plenty of plant-based fats and stay under 25 grams of carbohydrates, you will still use fat as an energy source. The difficulty is finding protein sources that are free of animal products and low in carbohydrates. Vegan protein replacements can be processed and refined with grains, which will cause a spike in glucose levels. Focusing on good healthy fats (avocado, coconut, nuts, and olive oil) while eating plenty of low-carb vegetables may work to get you into ketosis. Always watch your macros to ensure you meet your protein and fat goals.

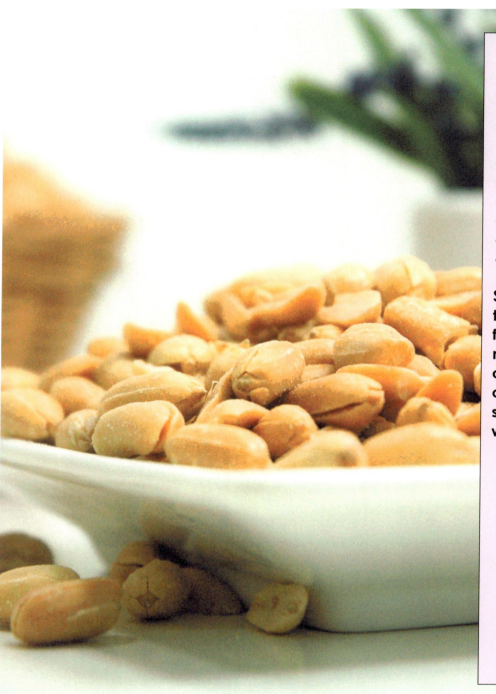

Our Best Loved Snack Options

- Pickles/Olives
- Cheese Stick
- Broccoli w/ Ranch
- Walnuts
- Hard Boiled Egg
- Avocado Slices
- Salami
- Cottage Cheese
- Zucchini sticks

Snacks are a great way to get high in healthy fats, but check your nutrition labels on all snacks for hidden carbohydrates to make sure you are staying within your macros!

7. How Do I Make Sure to Get Enough Fats?

Getting enough fat in your diet is essential to cross over into ketosis. Eating too many carbohydrates or even too much protein can stop your body from getting into that fat-burning metabolic state. Following this diet will allow you to hit these targets for all macros. If you struggle with getting enough fat into your diet in the future, consider adding in bulletproof coffee, and maybe even start taking a supplement like Caprylic Acid, an MCT oil.

8. The Role of Micronutrients?

Nutrition is more than just hitting your macronutrient goals for fat, protein and carbohydrates. Only eating fats and protein can be a very dangerous way to approach ketosis. Our bodies also need micronutrients like vitamins, minerals and electrolytes to survive. For example, even though a banana is high in carbohydrates, it has a lot of micronutrients in the form of potassium, magnesium and many b vitamins. Many of the micronutrients that we need come from fruits and vegetables, and since we are not eating many fruits, it is very important to eat nutrient-rich greens and to supplement with an electrolyte solution.

This Is NOT a Calorie Restricted Diet! Choose a healthy calorie count that is right for your height, weight and activity level. Eat when you are hungry! It is about the quality of nutrition, not about cutting the quantity.

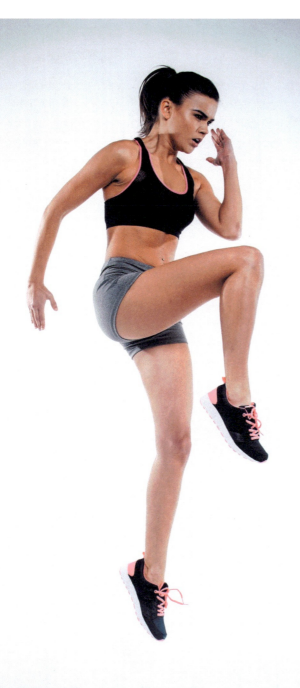

Ketogenic Eating & Metabolism

Your body can run off of either of these two fuel types, fats or sugars. Carbs (sugar) are processed by the liver, which then produces insulin to regulate the spike in blood sugar. However, fats are metabolized differently. When you consume fat instead of carbs, it does not affect your insulin production. During ketogenic eating, carbs/sugar are very restricted leaving fat as the fuel source, allowing your metabolism to regulate your body's insulin levels much more efficiently.

Keto Field Guide on Instagram!

Use our Hashtags!
#Ketofieldguide
#kfgchallenge #KFG

Medical Concerns

If you have a medical concern, definitely consult with your doctor about whether this is safe for you to consider, however I will say that many traditional doctors will not be on board with a high fat diet for various reasons. It will be up to you and your doctor to weight out the pros and cons. There is now more medial science than ever to support this type of eating style, so I urge you to do your homework and ask all the questions you have. Here are a few of the most commonly inquired about medical concerns and a quick guideline for each.

Should I Do Keto With:

1. Gastric Ulcers?

YES! Prescribed diets for gastric ulcers will exclude processed, refined foods and processed refined sugars, both of which are eliminated in the ketogenic diet. There is evidence that medium chain triglycerides (MTCs) heal and rebalance your gut with antimicrobial properties. You can find MTCs in our favorite supplement, Caprylic Acid, and in coconut oil.

2. Diabetes?

YES! Low carbohydrate diets are often prescribed by doctors to diabetic patients due to the low glycemic load and low insulin response. There is a danger in being too low in blood sugar for people with diabetes. Always make sure to talk to your doctor, know your numbers (and check them often), and never do strenuous exercise before bed. People with diabetes may choose to count net carbs instead of total carbs toward their 25g limit a day.

3. Kidney Issues?

YES! Kidneys do not metabolize fat, so people with kidney issues will not experience excess adverse effects. Consult with your doctor for any additional concerns related to kidneys.

4. Gastric Bypass?

YES! Low-carb diets are recommended for gastric bypass patients. However, your doctor may want you to stay on a different macronutrient count (higher in protein), so always consult with your medical team first. Consuming large amounts of fat can cause upset stomach and may make it difficult to get a sufficient amount of protein. It will take trial and error to get the correct percentages of macronutrients.

5. No Gallbladder or Fatty Liver Disease?

NO! Not recommended for ketosis, although I have coached people without gallbladders through ketosis successfully and with no issues. This is a disclaimer and it is entirely up to you and your health care professional to decide.

6. Hypertension?

Yes! But you may want to watch your salt intake. Some recipes have a large salt quantity and should be switched out for a lower sodium option. For example, Italian Chopped Salad in week one will not be suitable for a person with hypertension. Consider swapping this recipe out for any lunch recipe in week 2. Consider using a salt-free seasoning in place of salt in all other recipes.

Ketogenic Eating Has Been Prescribed For:
Epilepsy, Alzheimer's, Cancer, Diabetes

Lifestyle and Fitness

Besides the basics, the nutrition, and the medical concerns, you may be wondering about where you can bend the rules and how you can make this work for your current lifestyle. Here are a few tips from the most commonly asked question about lifestyle and fitness;

1. Can I Drink Alcohol?

There are low carbohydrate options if you want (need) to have an adult beverage during this time. Although it is not advisable, living a healthy life is all about balance. Spirits and liquors will have no carbohydrates on the label and can be consumed in small portions. Consuming too much of this will however produce an insulin response similar to eating sugar. Limit your intake to 1 drink, 3 times a week at the max. See our alcohol guide in the back of this book.

2. What is Keto Flu and How to Avoid It?

Keto Flu refers to the time it takes you to transition from using your carbohydrate energy system to using your fat energy system. This time is an adjustment that typically takes about 3-4 days. During this time, you are drastically decreasing your fruit intake and can lose electrolytes, which causes you to feel dehydrated or flu-like. Combat this process by taking an exogenous ketone supplement and drinking plenty of sugar-free electrolytes.

3. What can I Take Instead of my Workout Supplement?

Look for sugar-free versions of your current supplements first. BCAAs and other post-work out recovery supplements can be taken in pill form without the carbohydrates. To supplement your protein shake, focus on eating whole, high quality protein instead. If you are taking a pre-workout, bulletproof coffee can be a great substitution. You may also find that you don't need a pre-workout once you are in ketosis due to the increase in energy after the first 4 days.

4. Can I Exercise on Keto?

Yes! Depleting your muscle's energy storage of glycogen (sugar) by doing resistance exercises at the beginning of a keto challenge can be beneficial to get you into ketosis quicker. Ketosis is great for long and slow exercises, but very difficult for fast burst, muscle-building exercise. It is not advised to lift heavy on a strict ketosis diet.

5. Can I Gain Muscle on Keto?

It is not advised to set a muscle building goal on ketosis. There are athletes who are keto-adapted and can use the fat energy storage very efficiently; these people may be able to gain muscle on this diet. They accomplish this by cycling off keto macros during high intensity exercise and are usually already "keto Adapted". The increase in carbohydrates is utilized by the muscles, allowing the body to stay in overall ketosis. This is a difficult and very strict plan. Find our keto for bulkers plan at the back of this book.

If you would like to set a muscle building goal on ketosis, we recommend working with an SSOHealth coach

6. Are There Keto-Friendly Food Brands?

Food-label reading and macro tracking become very important during ketogenic eating. Be mindful of the carbohydrates hidden in spreads like mayo, ketchup, mustard, and salad dressings! Look at processed meats for added fillers and glazes. When at all possible, choose natural and simple foods like unprocessed meats and cheeses, nuts, eggs, and greens.

7. Can I Drink Diet Soda with a Ketogenic Diet?

Yes, you can enjoy a diet soda without kicking out of ketosis and while avoiding a spike in blood sugar. However, consuming artificial sweetened products does potentially increase your risk of GI inflammation and cancer. Many of these options like Splenda (Sucralose, aspartame) are chemical compounds that cannot be used as fuel in the body, and that is why they have zero calories. The irregular shape of the chemical compound in fake sugar does not stick or stack like natural sugar. Where natural sugar is a straight line, chemical sugar is more like a lightning bolt, causing it to act more like a free radical bumping into the lining of the blood vessels and causing damage. This theory is why chemical compounds like Splenda are linked to increased risk of cancer. Other options for sugar substitutes are sugar alcohols like the ones used in mouthwash (xylitol, Sorbitol, Erythritol). These are naturally occurring compounds, but they typically cause the same GI upset and inflammation in the gut. Choose naturally sweetened products over chemically sweetened products whenever possible.

8. Where do I Find Keto-friendly Recipes?

You are in luck! Keep reading to find two full weeks of ketogenic recipes created just for you! If you want access to even more recipes and support, consider joining the SSOHealth Keto E-Community all access program that includes access to our constantly growing keto Pinterest board, private YouTube Chanel, and private Facebook group. Find out more at www.ketofieldguide.com

Adjust your calorie intake for weight loss!

9. How do I Make Sure I am Getting the Right Amount of Calories?

Calorie needs will be different for each person. For most people, the 1800-1600 calorie diet will be perfect, but for others that may be too much or too little. Calorie needs are based on three factors: 1. Your current body weight, 2. Your activity level, and 3. Your goals. The higher your body weight and activity level, the higher your calorie need will be, especially if you are not looking to lose much weight. Review the calorie count for each day to help you decide if you need to modify intake. For greater weight loss or for smaller, less active people, skip the snacks and consider reducing portion sizes just slightly. For more active and higher calorie needs people, keep the snacks, double the snack options, or consider adding a dessert (like a fat bomb). If you are unsure of your calorie needs, consider working with an SSOHealth Coach for personalized programming.

10. Where do I Find More Information on Ketosis?

Check out our blog and get connected on our social media pages on Facebook, Instagram, and YouTube. Sign up for our keto newsletter for more information that is expertly curated for you regularly. Kick it up a notch with the KFG All Access E-Pass where you will get even more support and resources for your low-carb lifestyle! All of this is available at www.ketofieldguide.com.

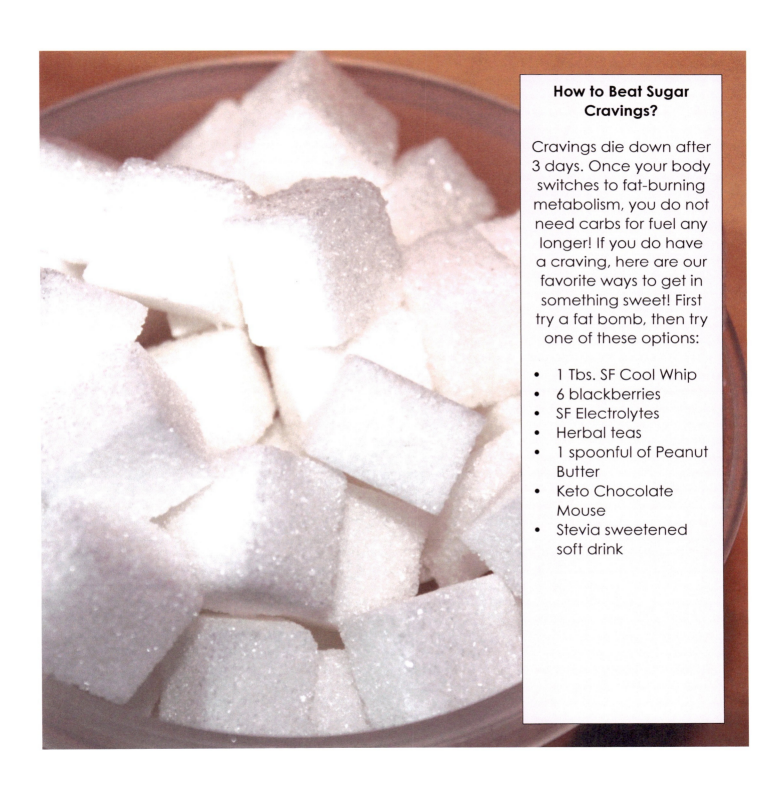

How to Beat Sugar Cravings?

Cravings die down after 3 days. Once your body switches to fat-burning metabolism, you do not need carbs for fuel any longer! If you do have a craving, here are our favorite ways to get in something sweet! First try a fat bomb, then try one of these options:

- 1 Tbs. SF Cool Whip
- 6 blackberries
- SF Electrolytes
- Herbal teas
- 1 spoonful of Peanut Butter
- Keto Chocolate Mouse
- Stevia sweetened soft drink

Ketogenic Field Guide
14-Day Meal Plan

Master Meal Plan Week 1

Day	Breakfast	Lunch	Snack	Dinner	Total Cals	Macros (F/P/C)		
1	BP Coffee + 3 Pancakes	Chicken Salad	String Cheese + 1/2 0z Walnuts	Meatballs Stirfry	1686	69%	5%	24%
2	BP Coffee + 3 Quiche Cups	Italian Salad	Cauliflower & Ranch + 1/2 0z pistachios	Chicken and Brussels	1722	70%	6%	22%
3	BP Coffee + 3 Pancakes	Chicken Salad	String Cheese + 1/2 0z Walnuts	Meatballs Stirfry	1686	69%	5%	24%
4	BP Coffee + 3 Quiche Cups	Italian Salad	Cauliflower & Ranch + 1/2 0z pistachios	Chicken and Brussels	1722	70%	6%	22%
5	BP Coffee + 3 Pancakes	Chicken Salad	String Cheese + 1/2 0z Walnuts	Meatballs Stirfry	1686	69%	5%	24%
6	BP Coffee + 3 Quiche Cups	Italian Salad	Cauliflower & Ranch + 1/2 0z pistachios	Chicken and Brussels	1722	70%	6%	22%
7	BP Coffee + 3 Pancakes	Chicken Salad	String Cheese + 1/2 0z Walnuts	Meatballs Stirfry	1686	69%	5%	24%

Master Meal Plan Week 2

Day	Breakfast	Lunch	Snack	Dinner	Total Cals	Macros (F/P/C)		
8	BP Coffee + 3 Egg Muffins	Buffalo Chicken Salad	Cauliflower & Ranch	Tacos	1783	65%	5%	22%
9	BP Coffee + Avocado Bagel	Loaded Burger	1/2 oz Walnuts	Asparagus Chicken	1882	68%	3%	22%
10	BP Coffee + 3 Egg Muffins	Buffalo Chicken Salad	Cauliflower & Ranch	Tacos	1783	65%	5%	22%
11	BP Coffee + Avocado Bagel	Loaded Burger	Cauliflower & Ranch + 1/2 0z pistachios	Asparagus Chicken	1722	68%	3%	22%
12	BP Coffee + 3 Egg Muffins	Buffalo Chicken Salad	Cauliflower & Ranch	Tacos	1783	65%	5%	22%
13	BP Coffee + Avocado Bagel	Loaded Burger	1/2 oz Walnuts	Asparagus Chicken	1882	68%	3%	22%
14	BP Coffee + 3 Egg Muffins	Buffalo Chicken Salad	Cauliflower & Ranch	Tacos	1783	65%	5%	22%

Note- Macro % don't add up to 100 because fiber is not reflected in this split

Grocery Shopping Guide

Grocery Shopping Tips!

1. Before you shop, check your pantry! You may already have some of these ingredients. This is especially true for week two! Week two items marked with an asterisk (*) are items you may have purchased in week 1 and likely will not need to purchase again but check the portion size just in case!
2. Portions: These grocery lists are enough to prepare four servings of each recipe for one week; however, some products may come in sizes larger than needed for one week. Items like nuts, lunch meat, and fresh mozzarella may be cheaper in 12 oz bulk. Purchase bulk and then portion out and freeze additional portions for later use.
3. Labels: check labels and choose products that are full fat and low-carbohydrate, striving for less than 1 carb per serving if at all possible. Choose low sodium options as available as well. Never choose fat free products.
4. Save Money: buy produce loose and unpackaged. This will save on packaging and will allow you to only get the amount you need for the week. Buy in bulk to double the recipe, cook for more than yourself, or to prep and freeze for future weeks.
5. Save Time: save a step on prep by buying packaged produce that is already sliced. Buy canned garlic, sliced mushrooms, pre-washed and cut greens, and pre-sliced onion. Save time in the grocery store by avoiding the inner isles, you will find almost everything you need on the outer perimeter of the store.
6. Swaps: Swap out spinach for kale if you can't find kale or prefer spinach. It will save you a few carbs but will cost you some fiber and vitamins. Swap out any spices for other spices you prefer or leave them out completely without changing the nutrients of the meal very drastically.

Week One Grocery Check-List

Pantry

- ☐ Ranch Dressing
- ☐ Baking Powder
- ☐ Cinnamon
- ☐ Stevia Drops
- ☐ Vanilla Extract
- ☐ Sugar-free Syrup
- ☐ Dijon Mustard
- ☐ Red Wine Vinegar
- ☐ Dried Oregano
- ☐ 16 oz Olive oil
- ☐ 1 jar Kalamata Olives
- ☐ 8 oz Mayonnaise
- ☐ 16 oz Beef Stock
- ☐ Chili Powder
- ☐ Onion Powder
- ☐ 2 oz Raw Walnuts
- ☐ 4 oz Pistachios
- ☐ Sugar-free Peanut Butter
- ☐ Parmesan Crisps

Deli

- ☐ 1/4 lb Salami
- ☐ 1/4 lb Ham

Produce

- ☐ 1 Green Bell Pepper
- ☐ 2 Bulbs Garlic
- ☐ 1 Red Onion
- ☐ 1 Bunch Cilantro
- ☐ 1 Bunch Celery
- ☐ 8 oz Mushroom
- ☐ 1 Large Head Broccoli
- ☐ 16 oz Brussel Sprouts
- ☐ 1 Lime
- ☐ 1 Head Romaine Lettuce
- ☐ 6 oz Bag Kale
- ☐ 2 Heads Cauliflower
- ☐ 1 Large Tomato
- ☐ 2 Cartons Blackberries
- ☐ 2 Avocados

Dairy

- ☐ 2 Dozen Eggs
- ☐ 1/2 Carton Heavy Cream
- ☐ 1 Box Unsalted Butter

Cheese

- ☐ 8 oz Cream Cheese
- ☐ 8 oz Shredded Cheddar
- ☐ 4 oz Fresh Mozzarella
- ☐ 10 Mozzarella cheese sticks

Meat

- ☐ 1 lb. Bacon
- ☐ 3 lb. Chicken Breasts
- ☐ 1 lb. Ground Beef (85% lean)

Week Two Grocery Check-List

Pantry

- ☐ 8 oz Olive oil*
- ☐ 5 oz Hot Sauce
- ☐ Blue Cheese Dressing
- ☐ Ranch Dressing*
- ☐ 8 oz Mayonaise *
- ☐ Beef Stock*
- ☐ 4 oz Sun-dried Tomatoes
- ☐ Italian Seasoning
- ☐ 1000 Island Dressing
- ☐ 7 oz Can Green Chili
- ☐ 4 oz Can Jalapeños
- ☐ 4 oz Walnuts
- ☐ 8 oz Almond Flour

Meat

- ☐ 3 lb. Chicken breast
- ☐ 2 lb. Ground beef
- ☐ 8 Breakfast sausage links
- ☐ 1 lb. Bacon

Produce

- ☐ 2 Yellow Onions
- ☐ 2 Bunches Spinach
- ☐ 8 oz Mixed Greens
- ☐ 1 Bulb Garlic
- ☐ 1 Cucumber
- ☐ 1 Lemon
- ☐ 1 Bunch Asparagus
- ☐ 2 Large Tomatos
- ☐ 1 Head Iceberg Lettuce
- ☐ 6 oz Sliced Mushrooms*
- ☐ 1 Head Cauliflower
- ☐ 2 Avocados

Dairy

- ☐ 1 Dozen Eggs
- ☐ 1 Box Unsalted Butter
- ☐ 8 oz Heavy Cream
- ☐ 4 oz Sour Cream

Cheese

- ☐ 8 oz Bag Shredded Cheddar
- ☐ 16 oz Shredded Parmesan Cheese
- ☐ 1 Pack Sliced Cheddar Cheese
- ☐ 8 Pack of String Cheese
- ☐ 8 oz Cream Cheese
- ☐ 8 oz Bag of Shredded Mozzarella *

Metabolic Journal

This section of the book is what sets our approach apart from other challenges or weight loss programs. Here you will be asked to reflect on your experience while you receive expert-level advice on what to expect and how to overcome usual obstacles. This is a great way to document and see the change that occurs in yourself over the days of the challenge. If you take the time to complete each day's activities, which I highly encourage and sincerely hope you do, you will likely have a better and more full experience. Each day you will be asked to rate your experience in three different categories; Energy, Mood, and Sleep (as measured by the previous night). You will give each category a number between 1-10 representing what you felt was the average for that day. 1 is the lowest and 10 is the highest or best score, so a score of 2 for "Energy" would be extremely low energy. A score of 8 for "Sleep" would indicate a relatively good night of rest during the previous night. We want to know how your body and mind reacts to the challenge of switching energy systems and we want you to track that trend through the 14-days to see how it changes. There are no right or wrong answers, just reflect honestly.

Each day you will also receive a "mindset makeover", or a small bit of inspiration to challenge your thinking. These themes go with what a persona would usually experience during the challenge on specific days. Again, this is is an example of how our approach differs from others, bringing more awareness into the challenge and allowing for more sustainable change to occur from the mind out to the body. I encourage you to take a few minutes to reflect on the message and maybe even jot a note or a few sentences down about what you are experiencing. What is alive in you at the moment that you read each day's makeover? If you plan to do this challenge quarterly with our group, this will be a fun thing to look back over and see how you change and grow each time.

In addition to these exercises, if you are testing your ketone output, make a star or dot on the page of the day that you first got into ketosis. If you slip up and kick out of ketosis, also mark a star or a dot on the day that you were kicked out and when you were able to return.

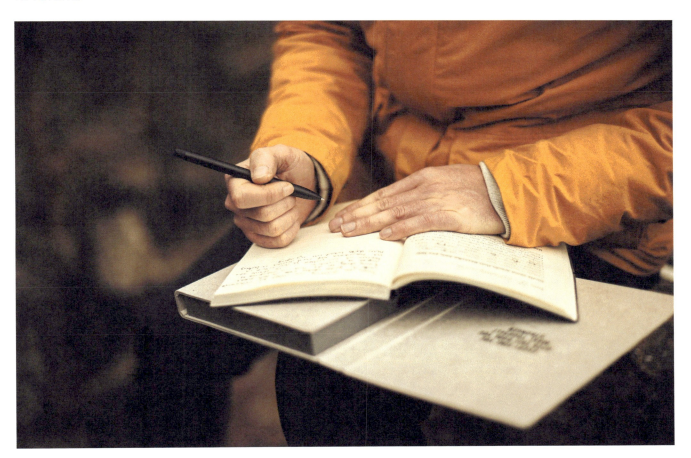

Creating A Mindset & Tracking Your Progress

Tracking your progress is a great way to keep motivated and to celebrate your successes. For additional ways to ensure success, follow these tips:

- Keep a journal of how you feel each day (Metabolic Journal section)
- Take a pre and post photo
- Take a pre and post waist measurement
- Keep track of your mental health changes and challenges
- Recognize that success comes in different forms
- Encourage others in your circle to join in to build your support system
- Connect to a community
    - Share your experience in our FB group
    - Share your favorite recipes
    - Ask questions and give advice from your own perspective

As you go into this 14-day challenge, begin to set an intention for what you want to accomplish. Ask yourself these questions:

1. Why am I doing this?
2. What do I hope to accomplish?
3. What barriers do I anticipate?
4. How can I reduce these barriers?
5. At the end of this challenge, I want to be:
6. After this challenge, I want to:

Now take a minute to document your current state so that you will have this baseline to compare at the end of this challenge.

Weight on Day 0:

Waist Circumference on Day 0:

Energy Level on Day 0:

Mental Clarity on Day 0:.

Welcome to Day 1!

Today I Feel:

Sleep:
1 2 3 4 5 6 7 8 9 10

Energy:
1 2 3 4 5 6 7 8 9 10

Mood:
1 2 3 4 5 6 7 8 9 10

Daily Macro Totals

1686 Calories
128 g Fat
106 g Protein
18.3 g Carbs

Calorie Count!
Remember to adjust your calorie consumption to your specific needs! Drop the BP coffee to reduce, or add a fat bomb to add calories, depending on your needs.

By now you should have:

- Purchased your food and meal prepped for week 1
- Purchased ingredients for bulletproof coffee and test strips
- Read through the FAQs
- Read through "Creating a Mindset" and set your goals
- Had your first coaching call to review your plan (Optional)

Today's Goals:

- ☐ Complete and document your weigh-in
- ☐ Test your ketone output
- ☐ Get active: 10-15 minute walk or activity of your choice
- ☐ Stay Hydrated: Drink at least 60 oz of purified water
- ☐ Find an accountability buddy: Tell someone about your new commitment and practice your knowledge on the topic by giving them some information

<u>Today's Mindset Makeover:</u>

You deserve to be healthy. You deserve to spend the money, time, and energy it takes to invest in yourself and your health, because you are worth it. Imagine if you treated your body like it belonged to someone you loved? How would that be different than what you are currently doing? Would you have more patience, more respect, and care for your physical body? In a world where we are taught to be so busy that we are not afforded time for self-care, be the person that prioritizes it. You are worth it. Your peace is worth it. Your health and your ability to use your body to experience life for many years to come depends on it.

Welcome to Day 2!
(The hardest day mentally)

What you might feel today:

- Tired, stomach upset, or headache
- Foggy feeling, low mood, or sugar cravings

Today's Goals:

- ☐ Test your ketone output
- ☐ Get active: Spend 10 minutes stretching
- ☐ Stay rested: Commit to more sleep tonight
- ☐ Find one success to celebrate: Recognize when you have passed up a food item that you would have normally eaten.

<u>Today's Mindset Makeover:</u>

Today is hard, but don't give up! You may feel like you need a sugar fix, but you really don't. Be mentally tough today. Tell yourself that the office doughnut or the afternoon cookie tray is poison, because you're not that far off. Sugar is inflammatory and addictive. You are working toward breaking that addiction. Honor your commitment to yourself. Our relationship with food is very complex. Not only is it vital for our survival, we also use food to make us feel happy, to celebrate with our loved ones, and to suppress negative thoughts or feelings. Congratulate yourself for taking steps toward a healthier relationship with food. Remember, you do not have to believe everything you think. Allow your mind to have the thoughts and feelings it has about this challenge, but then also let them pass. If you your brain is telling you that you "need" a small carb snack, observe that, validate it, and then let it pass.

Today I Feel:

Sleep:
1 2 3 4 5 6 7 8 9 10

Energy:
1 2 3 4 5 6 7 8 9 10

Mood:
1 2 3 4 5 6 7 8 9 10

Daily Macro Totals

1722 Calories
137 g Fat
96 g Protein
29 g Carb

Welcome to Day 3!
(The hardest day physically)

By now you should have:

- Conquered your day 2 sugar cravings
- Challenged your ideas on food wants vs needs
- Feel less bloated

Today's Goals:

- ☐ Complete and document your weigh-in
- ☐ Test your ketone output
- ☐ Get active: Move every joint in your body in every direction it can go- challenge your range of motion
- ☐ Don't give up: Recommit to your goals today
- ☐ Repeat after me: "My health is worth any discomfort or inconvenience I feel during this two-week challenge."

Today's Mindset Makeover:

Your body is like a sports car, it needs high grade specialized fuel to run and perform at its best. If you were to put mud or sludge into your sports car's gas tank, what would happen? Would you be surprised if the engine started to fail? We may spend time and money on our toys to keep them clean and running the best, but what about our bodies? When you choose your foods, think about what kind of fuel they will give you and the impact it will have on your body's ability to perform. High fat nutrition is premium 93 octane, while carbohydrates, specifically added processed sugars are way lower than 87. You wouldn't treat your sports car like that, why would you do that to your body?

Today I Feel:

Sleep:
1 2 3 4 5 6 7 8 9 10

Energy:
1 2 3 4 5 6 7 8 9 10

Mood:
1 2 3 4 5 6 7 8 9 10

Daily Macro Totals

1686 Calories
128 g Fat
106 g Protein
18.3 g Carbs

Welcome to Day 4!

By now you should have:

- Gotten into ketosis!! WOOHOO
- Start to feel less sluggish and more clear-minded
- Seen a little weight reduction (1-2 lb.)

You might feel:

- Backed up or constipated- add an extra serving of leafy greens, drop the cheese snacks, and get active
- Still have a lingering headache- hydrate with electrolytes (eat a few pickles).

Today's Goals:

- ☐ Test your ketone output
- ☐ Get active: 10-20 minutes of your favorite slow cardio
- ☐ Don't over think it: Feeling discomfort in your stomach is common and does not mean that something is wrong. Your body is still adjusting to this new diet, give it another day.

Today's Mindset Makeover:

Change is often difficult and painful. One way to reduce the pain of change is to understand it. One theory of change says that people fall into one of six categories of change; 1. Not ready to change, 2. Thinking about change, 3. Making preparations to change, 4. Beginning to change, 5. Have changed, 6. Continued in this change for over 6 months. Where are you at in your healthy change journey? It is probably a mix of change stages depending on the health change, and that is okay. Let's focus on changing nutrition habits. Where are you in your willingness to change nutrition habits permanently? Whatever that stage is, just begin to focus on getting to the next stage. If you are in the "thinking about change" stage, what would it take to get you to the "making preparations" phase? Take a minute to brainstorm what tools and support you would need to move up a level.

Today I Feel:

Sleep:
1 2 3 4 5 6 7 8 9 10

Energy:
1 2 3 4 5 6 7 8 9 10

Mood:
1 2 3 4 5 6 7 8 9 10

Daily Macro Totals

1722 Calories
137 g Fat
96 g Protein
29 g Carbs

Welcome to Day 5!

By now you should have:

- Adjusted to the new diet and have less gastric upset
- Have increased energy during the day
- Read through the FAQs again

Today's Goals:

- ☐ Test your ketone output
- ☐ Get active: 10-20 minutes of your favorite slow cardio
- ☐ Share your experience so far with someone

Today's Mindset Makeover:

Surrender is a part of moving into a new change. This will likely come in a few different forms. You may feel surrender to this diet, you may feel surrender to giving up a particular food that you "can't have" now. An important thing to note about surrender is that it is voluntary, unlike defeat. Surrender is making the harder choice and being completely at peace with it, even though it challenges you and maybe makes you feel bad in the short term. Find your peace of mind in the things you surrender or give up during the challenge. It's okay to feel sad or emotional about food, but practice moving into a surrender mindset where you actively choose not to have that food. Say to yourself "I can have this food, but I choose not to at this moment for the greater good of my health." Choosing not to indulge in the food of choice can be a way to claim power back over your choices. After all, you do have a choice, you always have a choice. Make this choice one that you can feel good about.

Today I Feel:

Sleep:
1 2 3 4 5 6 7 8 9 10

Energy:
1 2 3 4 5 6 7 8 9 10

Mood:
1 2 3 4 5 6 7 8 9 10

Daily Macro Totals

1686 Calories
128 g Fat
106 g Protein
18.3 g Carbs

Not Losing Weight?

Adjust your calories and consider intermittent fasting. Drop 200 Cals and only eat between 10 am and 5 pm

Welcome to Day 6!
(The hardest day socially)

If you started this journey on a Monday, you should now be going into your weekend! Get ready for a bumpy ride. Often times we are challenged harder during our weekends than we are during the work week, with diet traps and social events oh my! If you find yourself in a social bind, make sure to research keto-friendly options at any event or restaurant you will be eating at. Use our restaurant guide in the back of the book.

Today's Goals:

- ☐ **Test your ketone output**
- ☐ **Get active:** Challenge yourself with a longer walk or try another form of moderate cardio, shoot for 20-30 minutes
- ☐ **Stay the course:** Plan ahead for events and grocery shop for next week's meal prep.

Today's Mindset Makeover:

Love yourself through mistakes. Do not let one mistake ruin your challenge. Get back up and try again. There will be pitfalls, but they only define you if you choose to stay there. Commit to forgiving yourself for any mistakes and then let that ISH go! Move forward in your health with a determined mindset. Keeping with the sports car metaphor, think of making a mistake like blowing a tire. If you got a flat in one tire, you wouldn't immediately pull over and slash the rest of the tires because the one is flat. That would make getting to your destination impossible. Instead, you would work with the flat and get it fixed as soon as possible. Treat any mistakes the same way. Don't live in a bad decision, fix the flat and move forward.

Today I Feel:

Sleep:
1 2 3 4 5 6 7 8 9 10

Energy:
1 2 3 4 5 6 7 8 9 10

Mood:
1 2 3 4 5 6 7 8 9 10

Daily Macro Totals

1722 Calories
137 g Fat
96 g Protein
29 g Carbs

Welcome to Day 7!

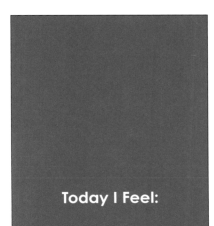

Today I Feel:

Sleep:
1 2 3 4 5 6 7 8 9 10

Energy:
1 2 3 4 5 6 7 8 9 10

Mood:
1 2 3 4 5 6 7 8 9 10

Daily Macro Totals

1686 Calories
128g Fat
106g Protein
18.3g Carbs

By now you should have:

- Seen more weight reduction (2-4 lb.)
- Felt less stiff in your joints
- Scheduled your next coaching call for some time soon (Optional)

Today's Goals:

- ☐ **Complete and document your weigh-in**
- ☐ **Test your ketone output**
- ☐ **Get active:** Spend time in a green space with fresh air
- ☐ **Take the progress survey:** Track your week one progress online, make sure to input your info before your coaching call so you can discuss with your coach (Optional)

Today's Mindset Makeover:

Let's get real. What is realism anyway? I would argue that being real takes courage and insight. You need to be able to challenge yourself to get out of your comfort zone, but you also need to do it in a way that creates positive forward motion, not crippling anxiety. When setting a goal, follow the SMART rule. Make sure that it is Specific, Measurable, Attainable, Realistic, and Time-based. Once you settle on a goal, also ask yourself these questions: Is it simple? Will it work? Can I do it? Will I do it? If you pass with all "yes" answers, then it is probably a realistic goal and you are free to get going on it. If not, rework it to make it more attainable, even if it is really simple. Find a realist goal to go into week two with today. Challenge yourself but be SMART about it.

Welcome to Day 8!

You made it through week one!
By now you should have:

- Completed your second coaching call
- Completed your week one results survey
- Purchased groceries and prepped week 2 meals

Today's Goals:

- ☐ **Complete and document your week two weigh-in**
- ☐ **Test your ketone output**
- ☐ **Get active:** Try some yoga stretching
- ☐ **Meditate on the process of your goals**

Today's Mindset Makeover:

Let's play devil's advocate. I want you to revel in your successes, but what if I told you that you should also not be too attached to your progress? Learning to let go of attachment to progress can be one of the most freeing things ever. Having a goal is great, but also dangerous. Not meeting a goal can be just as damaging as never setting a goal in the first place. Set the goal but value the work that it takes to get to the goal over the destination of the goal. Making this change is setting you up for a lifetime of better health, regardless if the scale moves or not. See if you can take the goals that you set for yourself and break them into smaller goals, ones you can check off immediately and ones that you can check off very soon. Set a course for achieving each goal, but let that course be as flexible and adaptable as it needs to be.

Today I Feel:

Sleep:
1 2 3 4 5 6 7 8 9 10

Energy:
1 2 3 4 5 6 7 8 9 10

Mood:
1 2 3 4 5 6 7 8 9 10

Daily Macro Totals

1783 Calories
165g Fat
73g Protein
19.4g Carbs

Welcome to Day 9!

By now you should have:

- Learned something about your body
- Learned something about your mind
- Learned something about nutrition and how it affects you
- Decided on if you are going to continue eating this way after the challenge ends

Today's Goals:

- ☐ **Test your ketone output**
- ☐ **Get active: Dance to a few songs on the radio**
- ☐ **Review week one Metabolic Journal records**

Today's Mindset Makeover:

Building on day 8 is the concept of stoicism. In stoicism, it is said that it is best to best in balance of emotion: not too happy and not too sad. If you notice yourself being too excited either way, work toward coming back into balance. If something bothers you, notice that. How can you feel the feeling of being bothered on a spectrum? Try to feel bothered but not to the point that it diminishes your peace of mind. Often times when we make a significant change and start to see success, we feel very passionately about it. There is danger here too, danger of making another big change too quickly, committing to an unrealistic goal, or doing too much of a good thing. If. You are feeling terrible about your challenge, find a way to make it more manageable. If you are feeling great about your challenge, stay the course and resist the urge to add another health change. The bottom line here is don't overdo it if you feel great, and don't quit if you feel terrible.

Today I Feel:

Sleep:
1 2 3 4 5 6 7 8 9 10

Energy:
1 2 3 4 5 6 7 8 9 10

Mood:
1 2 3 4 5 6 7 8 9 10

Daily Macro Totals

1882 Calories
165g Fat
73g Protein
19.4g Carbs

Welcome to Day 10!

By now you should have:

- Developed a baseline understanding of keto
- Came to terms with the fact that fat is not bad for you
- Decided on what works for you in this challenge and what doesn't

Today's Goals:

- ☐ **Test your ketone output**
- ☐ **Get active:** Try a yoga stretching program
- ☐ **Find a positive message to tell yourself and mean it**

Today's Mindset Makeover:

Self-talk and verbal communication matters immensely. You will practice and believe the things you think and say the most. How you phrase things and what you tell yourself matters. Your inner dialogue and how you treat yourself will likely influence your ability to thrive and reach your goals. Going back to the idea of treating yourself as if you were someone that you loved, think about how that would change your inner dialogue. Would you express more self-compassion? Can you be your biggest cheerleader? Can you ask yourself what it is that you need and then find a way to meet your own needs? If you lived in a perfect world and that one person that matters the most to you said the thing that you are longing to hear, what would that message be? Write that down and practice saying those exact words to yourself. Then, once you are comfortable with that, try actually meaning it when you say it.

Today I Feel:

Sleep:
1 2 3 4 5 6 7 8 9 10

Energy:
1 2 3 4 5 6 7 8 9 10

Mood:
1 2 3 4 5 6 7 8 9 10

Daily Macro Totals

1783 Calories
165g Fat
73g Protein
19.4g Carbs

Welcome to Day 11!

By now you should have:

- Tried out all of the recipes in the meal plan
- Had a very hard day and a very easy day
- Had a success and a failure
- Changed in some way

Today's Goals:

- ☐ **Test your ketone output**
- ☐ **Get active:** Test your balance with some standing yoga
- ☐ **Think about what is out of balance in your life and how to bring balance to that area**

Today's Mindset Makeover:

A great yoga teacher once told me that balance is new in every second. Balance is not something that you find once and you magically have for the rest of your life. Balance is a choice that is new each time. This is especially true in yoga standing poses. Balance is a second by second struggle to stay upright against the force of gravity in an unstable position. But our health and our life are like this also. Balance in your life and in your health will mean choosing the right path each time you have a choice, but it is complicated. Some days the right choice will be to push your limits, while other days the right or more balanced choice will be to rest. Some days a chocolate cake will be the most balanced breakfast while other days it will be a kale smoothie. If you are looking to master balance, all you need to know is that you can only ever master it in the moment. Practice your intuition and learn to listen to that above all else.

Today I Feel:

Sleep:

1 2 3 4 5 6 7 8 9 10

Energy:

1 2 3 4 5 6 7 8 9 10

Mood:

1 2 3 4 5 6 7 8 9 10

Daily Macro Totals

1882 Calories
165g Fat
73g Protein
19.4g Carbs

Welcome to Day 12!

By now you should have:

- Noticed a better sleep quality
- Noticed a stabilization in your mood
- Deviated from the meal plan successfully

Today's Goals:

- ☐ **Test your ketone output**
- ☐ **Get extra rest- take it easy**
- ☐ **Find something that makes you laugh**

Today's Mindset Makeover:

In order to succeed, you may need to be adaptable. Adaptability is necessary when you face an obstacle that your current plan will not allow you to face with success. This will be particularly helpful in social situations this weekend. Rather than being rigid or plastic, try being elastic. Bend and stretch when you need to, but always come back to your original form. Learning to adapt to a situation is much less anxiety-inducing than trying to maintain your position through a tough obstacle. Work smarter, not harder as the saying goes. Be creative in your problem solving, and always take a few deep breaths before making a decision. One weekend left, you got this!

Today I Feel:

Sleep:
1 2 3 4 5 6 7 8 9 10

Energy:
1 2 3 4 5 6 7 8 9 10

Mood:
1 2 3 4 5 6 7 8 9 10

Daily Macro Totals

1783 Calories
165 g Fat
73 g Protein
19.4 g Carbs

Welcome to Day 13!

By now you should have:

- A better understanding of what your calorie needs are while eating high fat nutrition
- A better understanding on how to balance a meal for Keto Macros
- Scheduled your challenge-end coaching call

Today's Goals:

☐ **Test your ketone output**
☐ **Don't cheat, you are almost there!**
☐ **Look up some new recipes**
☐ **Review KetoFieldGuide.com for more resources**

Today's Mindset Makeover:

Have you noticed a struggle over the past few days of this challenge? Struggle has a lot to teach us. When we struggle we tend to learn more about ourselves. Struggle teaches us more than harmony and balance ever will. If we are not struggling, we are not pushing our limits or striving for something new in our lives. Learn how to appreciate the struggle and find the lesson in it. What you struggle with often ends up being your biggest success and your life's mission. If you are struggling with this challenge, make sure to reach out to someone for support. Give life to the struggle instead of ignoring it. Share your struggles, you never know who else in your life may be struggling with a similar thing. Learn to lean on your community and adopt struggle as a natural part of the growth on your journey.

Today I Feel:

Sleep:
1 2 3 4 5 6 7 8 9 10

Energy:
1 2 3 4 5 6 7 8 9 10

Mood:
1 2 3 4 5 6 7 8 9 10

Daily Macro Totals

1882 Calories
165g Fat
73g Protein
19.4g Carbs

Welcome to Day 14!
(The finish line)

By now you should have:

- Felt really great about your progress
- Celebrated your successes
- Seen a little more weight loss (5+ lbs)
- Recommended cutting down on carbs to all of your friends
- Planned your first carb-filled cheat meal

Today's Goals:

- ☐ **Make it to the finish line**
- ☐ **Give yourself a High Five**
- ☐ **Read the "Now What" Section**

<u>Today's Mindset Makeover:</u>

As we approach the end of our challenge today, reflect on sustainability. What we have been doing in this challenge is not sustainable, nor should it be. This is meant to be an extreme change in your normal routine but is no good for the long term. What is able to be sustained over a long period of time will be the thing you are most likely to continue to do. Find a way to make healthy eating a sustainable practice. What lessons from this challenge will you adopt, which will you reject? What will sustainable health through nutrition look like for you and your family after this challenge? Anything extreme can only be sustained with great effort, but small changes that create lasting change can be sustained for years with flexibility and adaptability. Shift your mindset to the long-term future of health.

Today I Feel:

Sleep:
1 2 3 4 5 6 7 8 9 10

Energy:
1 2 3 4 5 6 7 8 9 10

Mood:
1 2 3 4 5 6 7 8 9 10

Daily Macro Totals

1783 Calories
165g Fat
73g Protein
19.4g Carbs

It's Day 15, Now What?!

Congratulations! You have survived 14 days with no added sugars and very little natural carbohydrates! Now that you have reached this milestone, let's take a minute to look back on your experience, and then look forward to where you will go next. Before we start, take a moment to revel in the fact that you did the challenge, regardless of whether you believe that you "passed" or 'failed", regardless of whether you achieved your desired outcome to the extent that you were hoping. Take a moment to recognize the mindset change, if any, that has happened.

Looking Back:

Go back and review your metabolic journal. Where did you feel low in energy? When did you get into ketosis (what day)? What days were the hardest? Easiest? And why? Did you find that you aligned with the typical feeling for each day as outlined in the journal? Was there something particularly impactful or inspiring that helped you along the way? What were your cravings like? Which foods did you crave and when? What helped you with cravings? Write these things down for future reference.

Looking Forward:

Now you will likely make your way back to a more balanced macro split while introducing carbohydrates back into your diet. If that is the case, what foods will you avoid, what foods will you cut out completely, and what will you allow yourself to reintroduce? If you are planning to stay in ketosis, how long will you go until your first cheat meal? How often will you have a cheat meal? What will it consist of? Are you planning to do this challenge again in a few months? If so, what will you do differently? What will you need to change or modify? Let the answers to these questions be your new commitment to yourself and to a healthier and more nutrition-based style of eating.

Want to keep going? Join us in the All Access E-Pass membership where we host a challenge just like this only with a network and community of supporters each quarter. To sign up for the KFG All Access E-Pass, go to www.ketofieldguide.com.

Measuring your Progress:

Weight Reduction:
Waist Reduction:
Change in Energy Level:
Change in Mental Clarity:

KFG All-Access E-Pass

What if you had a group of like-minded people who were there to help lift you back up whenever you wanted? If you have been toying around with the keto lifestyle and want to get more out of your hard work, this is for you.

The All-Access E-Pass gives you an invitation to be a part of a virtual community where people just like you are making healthy choices in their lives using high-fat nutrition. This is a great long-term solution to your busy and complex life.

What you get with the All-Access E-Pass:

Private Facebook Group

Our private Facebook group facilitates a community of keto challengers who can support and encourage others. This group will get a weekly tip and other helpful hints for the keto lifestyle. This private group is also where we will host and post about the quarterly challenge, post events and release special offers.

Private YouTube Chanel

Our private channel is full of video tutorials, education snippets, and product reviews. Includes how to set up your My Fitness Pal Macros and Calories, explications of keto principals, and walk-throughs of the quarterly challenges.

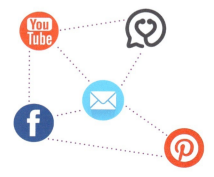

Private Pinterest Board

Our private Pinterest board is full of curated recipes for snacks, breakfast, lunch, dinner, desserts and drinks. This board is full of vetted and approved meal ideas and recipes guaranteed to keep you in ketosis while keeping your taste buds happy. Stop spending countless hours looking through recipes to find out if they are "really" keto friendly. There is a lot of misinformation out there, let us make it simple for you.

Quarterly Challenges

Hosted on the private FB page every quarter beginning in October, January, April, and July each year. This 14-day Challenge is a fun way to recommit to the healthy lifestyle and ban together with a group of keto challengers in the process. Participation in the challenge is free with the access pass but not mandatory. Participation will make you eligible to win prizes from SSOHealth!

Visit www.Ketofieldguide.com to get your All-Access E-Pass Now

Ketogenic Field Guide Recipes

Bulletproof Coffee

Ingredients

1 C. (8oz) Brewed Coffee
1Tbsp. Coconut Oil
1Tbsp. Unsalted Butter

Blend fresh hot coffee in the blender with coconut oil and butter on high for 20 seconds. Pour into your favorite mug and ENJOY!

224 Cals of High-Quality Fat

PRO TIPS:
- Use Filtered Water
- Use Organic Coffee
- Add a boost of exogenous ketones
- Never add sugar
- Use vanilla, cinnamon or cocoa to switch up the flavor

Bulletproof Coffee

Nutrition Facts
Servings: 1

Amount per serving

Calories	**221**
	% Daily Value *
Total Fat 25.2g	32%
Sodium 86mg	4%
Net Carbs 0g	0%
Protein .4g	

*% based on standard 2000 calorie diet, not on ketogenic diet recommendations.

Cream Cheese Pancakes

Ingredients

8 oz cream cheese
8 eggs
1 ½ tsp baking powder
1 ½ tsp cinnamon
1 ½ tsp stevia
1 ½ tsp vanilla

Toppings
½ C heavy cream
½ tsp stevia
1 tbs sugar-free syrup
Blackberries

Whipped Cream: Blend 1/2 c heavy cream in a blender until desired consistency, sweeten with stevia to taste. Set aside.

Pancakes: Blend remaining ingredients in a blender until smooth. Batter will be thin.

Preheat a non-stick skillet over medium heat. Grease skillet with butter or your favorite pan spray. Pour ½ of the mixture into the pan and cook for 2-3 minutes or until golden brown.

Carefully flip the pancake and cook for 1 additional minute.

Top with 1 tbs. whipped cream, 1 tbs. sugar-free syrup, and 4 berries.

Makes 4 servings:
1 serving = 3 pancakes

Cream Cheese Pancakes

Nutrition Facts
Servings: 1

Amount per serving	
Calories	429
	% Daily Value *
Total Fat 34.4g	44%
Sodium 361mg	16%
Net Carbs 9.6g	4%
Protein 15.5g	

% based on standard 2000 calorie diet, not on ketogenic diet recommendations.

Bacon & Kale Quiche Cups

Ingredients

10 eggs
1 lb bacon
3 C chopped kale
½ C diced tomato
½ C heavy cream
1 C shredded cheddar
1 tsp salt
Pepper to taste

Preheat pan over medium-high heat and preheat oven to 350. Add chopped bacon to preheated pan cook for about 4-5 minutes until fat renders and bacon starts to crisp. Add diced tomato, cook for 1 minute. Add chopped kale and cook for 1 additional minute until bacon is crisp and the vegetables are soft. Set aside to cool while preparing the eggs. Whisk or blend together eggs and cream until well blended, season with salt and pepper. Grease a 12-cup muffin tin with butter (or your favorite pan spray). Evenly distribute the bacon mixture among the muffin cups. Pour egg mixture into each muffin cup about ¾ of the way full. Top each cup with shredded cheddar. Bake in the oven for 15 minutes or until center of muffins are set.

Makes 12 individual cups
Serving Size: 3 cups

Bacon & Kale Quiche Cups

Nutrition Facts
Servings: 4

Amount per serving	
Calories	489
	% Daily Value *
Total Fat 36.2g	46%
Sodium 1204mg	52%
Net Carbs 7.2g	3%
Protein 32.8g	

% based on standard 2000 calorie diet, not on ketogenic diet recommendations.

Quick Chicken Salad

Ingredients

1 1/2 lb. chicken breast
½ c chopped celery
½ c chopped red onion
½ c chopped green bell
  pepper
½ c shredded cheddar
½ c mayonnaise
2 cloves minced garlic

Bake, grill, or boil chicken to preference. Dice cooked chicken into bite-sized pieces. Mix all ingredients in bowl and season with salt and pepper. Enjoy this alone, over a green salad, or in a lettuce wrap.

Makes 4 serving
Serving Size: *1/4 of the recipe (about 3/4 cup of mix and 2 lettuce leaves per serving).*

Quick Chicken Salad

Nutrition Facts
Servings: 4

Amount per serving
Calories   441

	% Daily Value *
Total Fat 28.8g	37%
Sodium 168mg	16%
Net Carbs 2.1g	1%
Protein 40g	

% based on standard 2000 calorie diet, not on ketogenic diet recommendations.

Quick Italian Chopped Salad

Ingredients

8 Cs chopped Romaine
4 oz (¼ lb.) ham
4 oz (¼ lb.) salami
4 oz (¼ lb.) fresh
    mozzarella
1 C kalamata olives
¼ C olive oil
2 Tbsp. red wine vinegar
1 tsp. dried oregano
2 cloves minced garlic
1 Tbsp. Dijon mustard
1/4 tsp salt
Pepper to taste

Vinaigrette Dressing:
Whisk together minced garlic, red wine vinegar, dried oregano, and Dijon mustard until combined. Slowly whisk in olive oil and season with salt and pepper.

Salad Construction:
Chop ham, salami, and mozzarella into bite size pieces (cubes or strips). Mix meat, cheese, and olives with vinaigrette. Store mixture and romaine separately, mix when you are read to eat. portioned out into 4 servings for quick grab-and-go lunches.

Makes 4 servings
Serving Size: *1/4 of the recipe (about 1 cup of mix and 2 cups of lettuce per serving*

Italian Chopped Salad

Nutrition Facts
Servings: 4

Amount per serving	
Calories	355
	% Daily Value *
Total Fat 30g	38%
Sodium 1394mg	61%
Net Carbs 9.6g	4%
Protein 16.7g	

*% based on standard 2000 calorie diet, not on ketogenic diet recommendations.

Meatball Stirfry

Ingredients

1 lb. ground beef
2 eggs
1 Avocado
1/3 C crushed parmesan
   crisps
2 cloves garlic
2 Tbsp. olive oil
1 C sliced mushrooms
2 C broccoli florets
1 C sliced green bell
   peppers
1 C beef stock
1 Tbsp. butter
1/2 cup shedded cheese
1 tsp salt
Pepper to taste

Combine ground beef, parmesan crisps, onion powder, minced garlic, and eggs in a medium bowl. Season with salt and pepper. Roll mix into golf ball sized portions (2 tablespoons of mix) . Preheat large sauté pan over medium heat. Add olive oil and sear meatballs until browned on all sides. Remove meatballs and set aside. Reduce heat to medium heat, add mushrooms, bell peppers and broccoli florets to the pan and cook for 2-3 minutes. Add beef stock to pan, scraping the bottom to lift anything that has stuck. Bring the liquid to a simmer, then add meatballs and cook for 5-7 minutes until cooked through and the stock has reduced. Remove from heat, add butter and stir constantly until melted and sauce thickens slightly. Sprinkle cheese over mix and let sit until melted. Serve with 1/2 of an avocado, sliced.

Makes 4 serving: 18 meatballs
Serving Size: 1/4 of recipe,
Approx. 4 meatballs per serving

Meatball Stir-fry

Nutrition Facts
Servings: 4

Amount per serving	
Calories	417
	% Daily Value *
Total Fat 24.5g	31%
Sodium 326mg	16%
Net Carbs 4.6g	2%
Protein 41.6g	

% based on standard 2000 calorie diet, not on ketogenic diet recommendations.

Chili Lime Chicken & Roasted Brussels

Ingredients

Chicken
1 1/2 lb. chicken breast
2 Tbsp. olive oil
1 Tbsp. chili powder
2 cloves mince garlic
1 Tbsp. lime zest
1 C beef stock
2 Tbsp. butter
2 Tbsp. chopped cilantro
1 tsp salt

Brussels
16 oz Brussels sprouts
2 Tbsp. olive oil
2 cloves minced garlic
S&P to taste

Mashed Cauliflower
6 oz chopped cauliflower
2 tablespoons butter
S&P to taste

Chicken: Cut chicken into strips and coat evenly with olive oil. In a bowl, combine chili powder, lime zest, garlic, and salt; rub evenly onto strips. Preheat skillet over medium heat. Sear strips in pan 2 minutes each side. Add beef stock and reduce heat, cover and simmer for 8 minutes or until chicken is cooked through. Remove from heat and stir in butter until melted. Top with chopped cilantro to serve.

Brussels Sprouts: Preheat oven to 375 F. Toss all ingredients in bowl to coat evenly. Place Brussels on lightly greased sheet tray. Bake for 8-10 minutes or until lightly browned and tender.

Mashed Cauliflower: Chop and boil cauliflower until tender. Drain well. Whip cauliflower in blender with salt, pepper, and butter.

Makes 4 serving:
Serving Size 1/4 of the recipe:
*Approx. 2 strips, 3/4 cup Brussels
And 2 tablespoons of mash.*

Chili Lime Chicken & Sides
Nutrition Facts
Servings: 4

Amount per serving	
Calories	491
	% Daily Value *
Total Fat 30.7g	39%
Sodium 425mg	18%
Net Carbs 8.7g	4%
Protein 42g	

% based on standard 2000 calorie diet, not on ketogenic diet recommendations.

Southwest Egg Muffins & Sausage Links

Ingredients

8 large eggs
2 tbsp. heavy cream
2 oz cream cheese
4oz green chili
1 C wilted spinach (2 cups chopped)
1/2 C shredded cheddar
1 tsp salt
Pepper to taste
8 sausage links

Preheat oven to 350. Drain all excess liquid from green chilies. Whisk or blend together eggs, green chili, cream cheese, cream, spinach, salt, and pepper until well blended. Grease a 12-cup muffin tin with butter (or your favorite pan spray). Pour egg mixture into each muffin cup until ¾ of the way full. Top each cup with shredded cheddar. Bake in the oven for 15 minutes or until center of muffins are set.

While cups are baking, brown all links in a skillet, then set aside to cool.

Makes 12 individual cups
Serving Size: 2 cups and 2 sausage links

Southwest Egg Muffins & Sausage links

Nutrition Facts

Servings: 4

Amount per serving	
Calories	356
	% Daily Value *
Total Fat 27.7g	36%
Sodium 1243mg	54%
Net Carbs 4.5g	2%
Protein 21.5g	

% based on standard 2000 calorie diet, not on ketogenic diet recommendations.

Jalapeño Bagel with Avocado Mash

Ingredients

2 cups Mozzarella
cheese grated
2 oz Cream cheese
1 cup Almond flour
1 teaspoon baking
powder
4 Tbsp. canned Jalapeno
2 Eggs
1 oz Cheddar
cheese grated
1/2 Avocado
1 tsp. Lemon Juice

Bagels:

Preheat oven to 400. Drain excess liquid from canned Jalapeño. Mix almond flour, baking powder, and jalapeño. Fold in eggs. In another bowl mix mozzarella and cream cheese. Microwave on medium until melted and smooth. Stir in almond flour mix a little at a time, then kneed with your hands until dough forms. Divide dough into 6 pieces. Form each peace into a round on the baking sheet. Sprinkle with cheddar cheese and bake for 25 minutes or until golden brown.

Avocado Mash:

Slice avocado and reserve 1/2 for future use. Mash 1/2 avocado with 1 teaspoon lemon juice. Top bagel with avocado mash, sprinkle with salt and pepper.

Makes 6 Bagels:
Serving Size 1 bagel

Jalapeno Bagel & Mashed Avocado

Nutrition Facts

Servings: 6

Amount per serving	
Calories	364
	% Daily Value *
Total Fat 30.7g	39%
Sodium 433mg	19%
Net Carbs 4g	3%
Protein 15g	

*% based on standard 2000 calorie diet, not on ketogenic diet recommendations.

Buffalo Chicken Salad

Ingredients

1.5 lb. chicken breast
1 Tbsp. olive oil
5 oz hot sauce
4 Tbsp. butter
1 C chopped cucumber
8 Tbsp. blue cheese
    dressing
1 C shredded cheddar
4 Cs mixed greens

Preheat pan with olive oil over medium heat. Season chicken breasts with salt and pepper, then brown on both sides. Remove chicken from pan and add hot sauce. Reduce heat to simmer. Whisk in butter until combined. Slice chicken into bite sized strips and then add back to pan. Cover and simmer for 6-7 minutes or until chicken is cooked through. Allow chicken to cool, then serve over mixed greens and top with cucumbers, cheddar, and blue cheese dressing. Package 4 portions of chicken and cheese separately from 4 portions of lettuce, cucumbers and dressing for quick grab and go lunches.

If buffalo sauce is too spicy, add more butter

Makes 4 serving:
Serving Size: 1/4 of the recipe

Buffalo Chicken Salad

Nutrition Facts

Servings: 4

Amount per serving	
Calories	549
	% Daily Value *
Total Fat 37.1g	48%
Sodium 1672mg	73%
Net Carbs 5g	3%
Protein 45.8g	

% based on standard 2000 calorie diet, not on ketogenic diet recommendations.

Loaded Bacon Cheeseburgers

Ingredients

1 lb. ground beef
1 lb bacon
1 medium onion sliced
8 slices of tomato
8 iceberg leaves
    separated
4 slices cheddar
2 Tbsp. butter
Thousand island dressing

Preheat oven to 350. Lay bacon out on baking sheet and bake until crispy, about 15 minutes. Preheat skillet on medium heat, add butter and sliced onions, cook for 10-15 minutes or until soft and caramelized. Separate ground beef into 4 equal patties (4 oz each). Season with salt and pepper and fry or grill to your desired temperature. Top each burger with onions and one slice of cheddar. Allow cheddar to melt and then let burger cool. Package each burger with 1 piece of bacon, 2 lettuce leaves, 2 tomato slices and a tablespoon of Thousand Island dressing.

Makes 4 serving:
Serving Size 1/4 of the recipe

Loaded Burgers

Nutrition Facts
Servings: 4

Amount per serving

Calories	669
	% Daily Value *
Total Fat 49.3g	63%
Sodium 744mg	32%
Net Carbs 3g	1%
Protein 50.4g	

% based on standard 2000 calorie diet, not on ketogenic diet recommendations.

Crispy Cheese Shell Tacos

Ingredients

Beef
1 lb. Ground Beef
1 tsp chili powder
2 cloves minced garlic
1/2 C sliced onion
1/2 tsp Salt
Pepper to taste

Topping:
(enough for 3 tacos)
1/4 C sliced tomato
1/2 C shredded lettuce
2 tbs. mayonnaise

Shells:
(makes 3)
1 1/2 C parmesan cheese

Preheat skillet over medium heat. Brown ground beef in skillet with onion, olive oil, garlic, chili pepper, salt and pepper. Once browned, set aside. Keep 1/4 of beef mixture out and put the rest in a container for later use. In a bowl, combine sliced tomato, lettuce and mayonnaise and set aside. Fill shells evenly with beef and topping to serve.

Shells:
With skillet still on medium heat, add 1/2 cup shredded parmesan cheese to the middle of the skillet in an even circular shape. Allow cheese to melt and then crisp before attempting to flip, about 90 seconds. Flip carefully and then brown on opposite side, about 40 seconds. Once both sides are browned, remove shell from pan and hang over a wire rack to cool into a taco times for 3 shells.

Makes 4 servings
Serving Size: 3 Tacos

Cheese Shell Tacos

Nutrition Facts
Servings: 4

Amount per serving	
Calories	**564**
	% Daily Value *
Total Fat 30.2g	39%
Sodium 1698mg	74%
Net Carbs 6.5g	3%
Protein 63.3g	

% based on standard 2000 calorie diet, not on ketogenic diet recommendations.

Creamy Asparagus Chicken

Ingredients

1.5 lb. chicken breast
2 Tbsp. olive oil
¾ C heavy cream
½ C beef stock
½ C sun-dried tomatoes
   chopped
1 C spinach chopped
3 cloves minced garlic
½ C shredded parmesan
   cheese
1 tsp. Italian seasoning
2 Cs asparagus chopped
2 Cs mushrooms,
   chopped

Preheat pan with olive oil over medium heat. Brown chicken breasts on both sides. Removed chicken from pan, add minced garlic, mushrooms, asparagus, sun-dried tomatoes and Italian seasoning, cook for 1-2 minutes (deglaze the pan with a splash of water if necessary). Add chicken stock and heavy cream, bring to simmer. Whisk in parmesan cheese until melted and smooth. Season with salt and pepper as needed. Add chicken back to pan, cover and simmer for 5-6 minutes. Add spinach, cover and cook for an additional 1-2 minutes or until chicken is cooked through.

Makes 4 serving:
Serving Size 1/4 of the recipe

Creamy Asparagus Chicken

Nutrition Facts

Servings: 4

Amount per serving	
Calories	538
	% Daily Value *
Total Fat 30.9g	40%
Sodium 176mg	59%
Net Carbs 9g	3%
Protein 56.5g	

*% based on standard 2000 calorie diet, not on ketogenic diet recommendations.

Dessert & Fat Bomb Snack Options

Peanut Butter Cheesecake Bites

Ingredients

4 oz. Cream Cheese softened
3/4 cup peanut butter
2 tbs. butter
3/4 cup almond flour
1/8 tsp. Vanilla Extract
8 drops Stevia

Blend all ingredients until smooth. Roll into bite-sized balls and store in the freezer.

Makes 12 serving
Serving Size: 1 piece

Peanut butter Cheesecake Bites
Nutrition Facts
Servings: 1

Amount per serving
Calories 156

% Daily Value *

Total Fat 14.2g | 18%
Sodium 116mg | 5%
Net Carbs 2.7g | 1%
Protein 5.1g

*% based on standard 2000 calorie diet,

Keto Chocolate Mousse

Ingredients

1 Medium Avocado
1/4 C. Baking Cocoa
8 oz. Cream Cheese
1/4 C. Heavy Cream
1/8 tsp. Vanilla Extract
8 drops Stevia

Pit and chop avocado. Add all ingredients to a blender and blend until smooth.

Makes 8 serving:
Serving Size 1/8 of the recipe

Keto Chocolate Mousse

Nutrition Facts
Servings: 1

Amount per serving
Calories 122

% Daily Value *

Total Fat 11.6g | 15%
Sodium 5mg | 0%
Net Carbs 21.6g | 1%
Protein 1.6g

*% based on standard 2000 calorie diet, not on ketogenic diet recommendations.

*Note: Ingredients for desserts are not reflected on the grocery list

Additional
Ketogenic Guides

No-Cook Busy/Lazy Keto Options

If you identify with me on being very busy and having limited time to prepare meals, you might do better with this no-cook, simple and quick recipe guide. This guide requires that you eat the same exact meal for 5 days straight. If you can handle that, I promise this will get you into ketosis with the minimal amount of effort possible. The top boxes represent your five-day grocery list for the busy work week. Try a few of the other recipes from the book for your weekend meals when you have more time!

Breakfast

- ☐ 8oz Coconut Oil
- ☐ 1 stick of butter
- ☐ Ground Coffee
- ☐ 3 avocados
- ☐ Pre-cooked bacon

Meal prep:

Prepare bulletproof coffee each am (Blend hot coffee with 1 tsp each coconut oil and butter) and enjoy on the way to work

Microwave bacon and toss it into a container with 1/2 an avocado, enjoy at mid-morning.

Totals for the day:
1300 Cals
97 g Fat
79 g Protein
28 g Carbs

Lunch

- ☐ 5 packs of tuna
- ☐ Kale salad mix
- ☐ Shredded parmesan
- ☐ Sugar free Cesar Salad dressing
- ☐ Walnuts
- ☐ 2 ct. Blackberries
- ☐ Low-carb protein powder

Meal prep:

Salad: Combine 1 pack of tuna and 1/2 cup kale with 1 tbsp. each cheese, dressing and walnuts in a container and enjoy at lunchtime.

8 oz of water or SF tea

Snack: berries & 1 scoop protein shake

Dinner

- ☐ 1 Rotisserie Chicken
- ☐ Sugar Free ranch
- ☐ Baby bell Cheese
- ☐ 10 oz bag of broccoli
- ☐ 10 oz bag of cauliflower
- ☐ Jar of pickles

Meal prep:

Heat and serve 4 oz of chicken with baby bell cheese melted over it

Dip broccoli and cauliflower in ranch to your hearts content.

Have a pickle, they have tons of electrolytes~!

Fast Food/Restaurant Keto Options

You may find yourself in need of an option at a restaurant. You should feel confident and happy about the choices you make when eating socially. You should be able to celebrate with your loved ones and still keep your nutrition goals. Here are a few options that will work in a pinch or a bind.

Breakfast

- ☐ Bacon and eggs
- ☐ Chorizo and eggs
- ☐ Steak and eggs
- ☐ Smoked salmon with cream cheese and vegetables
- ☐ Omelet with greens and cheese
- ☐ Coffee with heavy cream

Watch out for:
Potatoes, sauces, fruit. Sauces are often thickened with flour and places tend to sneak potatoes into everything. Omelets may even have flour to thicken.

Lunch

- ☐ Bun-less burger and side salad (ranch or Caesar)
- ☐ Full salad with bacon, blue cheese, chicken, avocado and ranch
- ☐ Dry rubbed grilled wings

Watch out for:
Salad dressings and marinade; Vinaigrettes and BBQ sauces are usually sweetened.

Dinner

- ☐ Any grilled protein with side of vegetables
- ☐ Ribs no sauce
- ☐ Steak with blue cheese
- ☐ Seafood (salmon, crab, lobster, fish, shrimp) in butter sauce

Watch out for:
Sauces and starchy vegetables. Choose green vegetables like broccoli, spinach, Kale, Brussels sprouts, and asparagus.

> 3 carbs a serving keto-Friendly Alcohol choices

- ☐ Vodka/Gin + Soda water + lime
- ☐ Skinny Kentucky Mule (Bourbon, SF ginger ale, lime)
- ☐ Champaign
- ☐ Dirty Martini (Vodka, Vermouth, Olive Juice)

SSO Sangria

- – 3 oz Pinot Grigio
- – 3 oz low-carb Kombucha (<5 g)
- – Squeeze of lemon

94 Cals, 7 carbs

Vegetarian Keto Options

It is possible to be vegetarian on a ketogenic diet as long as you hit those macro targets of 70% or higher in fats and 5% or lower in carbohydrates. If you choose to substitute a meat for a vegetarian product, be sure to check the labels for carbohydrates! Check out these modified recipes suitable for vegetarians!

Breakfast

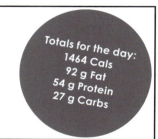

Totals for the day:
1464 Cals
92 g Fat
54 g Protein
27 g Carbs

Bulletproof Coffee
    And
Modified Quiche Cups
    Leave out the bacon and prepare as directed.
    Adjusted macros: 260 Cals, 7 g fat, 7 g protein, .5 g carbs

Lunch

Rustic Cob Salad
    Mix 1 cup Romain lettuce, 1/4 c tomato, 1/4 c cucumber, 1 hardboiled egg, 1 0z walnuts, 1/2 avocado and top with Sugar-free Ranch dressing.
    Adjusted Marcos: 436 Cals, 35 g fat, 14 g protein, 15 g carbs
Vegan Protein Shake (1 scoop Garden of Life Sport + 1 Tbsp. heavy cream)
    Macros: 136 Cals, 7 g fat, 15.3 g. Protein, 4.5 carbs,

Dinner

Tofu and veggies (Modified meatballs recipe)
    Sub in tofu (1/2 block = 1 serving) and veggie stock, + 1 tbsp. butter and 4oz Swiss
    Adjusted Marcos: 408 Cals, 18 g fat, 18 g protein, 7 g carbs
OR
Creamy Tempeh and asparagus (modified chicken recipe)
    Sub in Tempeh (1/4 cup = 1 serving) and veggie stock for chicken stock
    Adjusted Macros: 486 Cals, 40.5 g fat, 20 g protein, 13 g carbs

Bulkers Guide to Gaining Muscle in Ketosis

Gaining muscle on ketosis is a bit tricky. The system that allows muscles to hypertrophy, or increase in size, is the carbohydrate energy system. Muscles do need sugar to convert into energy to do the heavy lifting that is required to increase size. While that is a strict no go for ketosis, there are ways to get around it. Once your body is used to the fat for fuel energy system of ketosis, it may be easier to switch back and forth between the two systems with less and less lag time. There is also a theory that says there is a way to give your muscles just enough carbohydrate energy to get through a heavy lifting work out without spiking your insulin levels and kicking you out of ketosis. The theory says that if you take between 20-24 grams of carbohydrates in an immediately available form (like Gatorade or another liquid) right before a workout, the carbohydrates will be burned off before the liver needs to metabolize it. Using this theory, I have constructed a "Keto Adapted" 8-week program for heavy lifters who want the benefits of both ketosis and muscle gain. This is a very specific program design that requires calculations and strict adherence to varying diet programming. It is just as hard to set up as it is to follow, but the results are worth it for many people. Be warned, what you are about to read can be overwhelming.

If you have trouble setting up your goals, contact SSOHealth for custom programming.

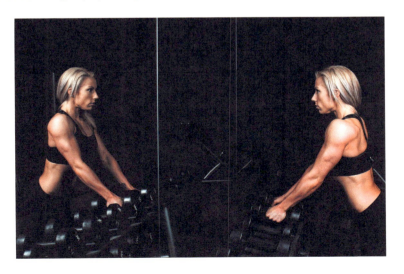

3-Step Process for Setting up Macros to Gain Muscle on Keto

Step 1- Set your calorie intake using your metabolic rate

- Calculate Basil Metabolic Rate (BMR), which is the number of calories you need to sustain your current weight
- Account for high activity level; add 1000 Cals for high activity level
- Account for desire to increase mass; add 350 Cals to activity adjusted BMR to arrive to your bulking calorie need
- EX Male: weight = 180 lb. (81.6 kg), Height = 5 ft '8 (172 cm) Age = 30 BMR = 1,746 Bulking Calorie Need = 1746 + 1000 + 350 = **3096**

BMR Calculations:

<u>**Male**</u> = 10 x weight (kgs) + 6.25 x height (cm) - 5 x age (years) + 5
<u>**Female**</u> = 10 x weight (kgs) + 6.25 x height (cm) - 5 x age (years) -161

Step 2- Set your macro split using your calorie intake target

- <u>Set up your macro split;</u> Macronutrients are categorized into Fat, Protein, and Carbohydrates. A typical keto macro split is 5/75/20 (C/F/P). Using the above calorie intake, the macro split will look like this:
  - Carbs = 3096(.05) = 154.8 Cals
  - Fat = 3096(.75) = 2322 Cals
  - Protein = 3096(.20) = 619.2 Cals
- <u>Vary your macro split;</u> You will notice on the bulker's guide to ketosis table below that macro percentages fluctuate depending on the type of exercise you are doing that day. This is very important. You must consume more carbohydrates at the right times on the right days or you will not get the results you are looking for.
- <u>Break your protein</u> into grams for ease using the Macros in grams conversions: 619.2/4 = 154.8 grams

Macros conversions: Grams to calories
- **Carbs** = 1 gram = 4 Cal
- **Fat** = 1 gram = 9 Cal
- **Protein** = 1 gram = 4 Cal

Step 3- Plan out your splits to match up to your exercise days

- Day 1- Normal keto macro split (5/75/20) + Lift heavy to expend all carbs stored in muscles
- Days 2-3 - Normal keto macro split and light exercise to allow your body to adapt to ketosis
- Day 4 - Protein modified keto macro split (10/60/30) + 25 grams of straight CHO (liquid carbs) immediately prior to high intensity and heavy lifting day (similar to cross-fit structure). Should exercise within 10 minutes of taking liquid CHO so that the liver never has to process the sugar.
- Days 5-22: Modified splits based on exercise
  - Light lift day- 10/60/30
  - Heavy lift day- 10/60/30 + 25g Liquid CHO
  - Cardio day- normal keto split 5/75/20
- Weeks 4-8: New adapted calculation for bulking during cross training days
  - Total Target Calorie Intake = 16 x desired body weight (190) = **3040 Cals**
  - Protein = 1lb/1gram = 190 grams of protein = 760 Cals (25%)
  - Fat = 30% = 3040(.3) = 912 Cals
  - Carbs = 45% = 3040(.40) = 1368 Cals

Sample splits for 8-week bulker's program

WK	M	T	W	TH	F	S	Sun
1	Lift Heavy + 5/75/20	Light Cardio + 5/75/20	Light Cardio + 5/75/20	Crosstrain + 10/60/30 + 25g CHO pre + BCAAs post	Lift light + 10/60/30	Light Cardio + 5/75/20	Crosstrain + 45/30/25
2-3	Lift light + 10/60/30	Light Cardio + 5/75/20	Lift light + 10/60/30	Crosstrain + 10/60/30 + 25g CHO pre + BCAAs post	Lift light + 10/60/30	Light Cardio + 5/75/20	Crosstrain + 45/30/25
4-8	Lift Heavy + 10/60/30 + 25g CHO pre + BCAAs post	Light Cardio + 5/75/20	Crosstrain + 45/30/25	Lift Heavy + 10/60/30 + 25g CHO pre + BCAAs post	Off + Cheat Meal	Lift Heavy + 10/60/30 + 25g CHO pre + BCAAs post	Crosstrain + 45/30/25
	Examples of Crosstraining: Cross-fit, rock climbing, intense hike, >20 min HIIT, swim, road bike, above moderate cardio (running, cycling, intervals, stairs, cardio-row)						

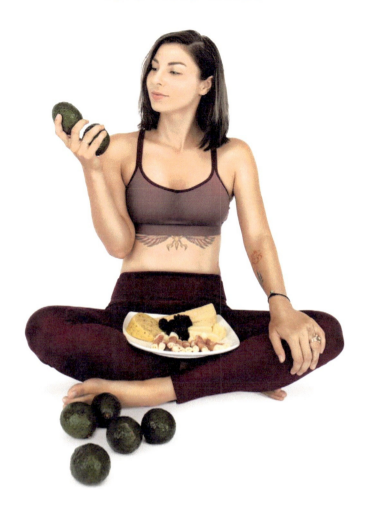

The addition of ketogenic eating has greatly improved my health and the health of the clients I serve. I hope you find the same amazing benefits in your life. I hope you take your new-found health and use it to live your best life. Go! Explore! Be present! Take the trip! Experience life! Connect deeply with the people around you and with your community! Be an inspiration to someone you know! Be a success story, because you deserve to be healthy and you are worth it!

- XOXO, Brea